Far Infrared Magnesiu

Pure Nature Cures School
of Mineral & Spa Therapies

Far Infrared Magnesium Wrap Course

For Clinic & Home Use

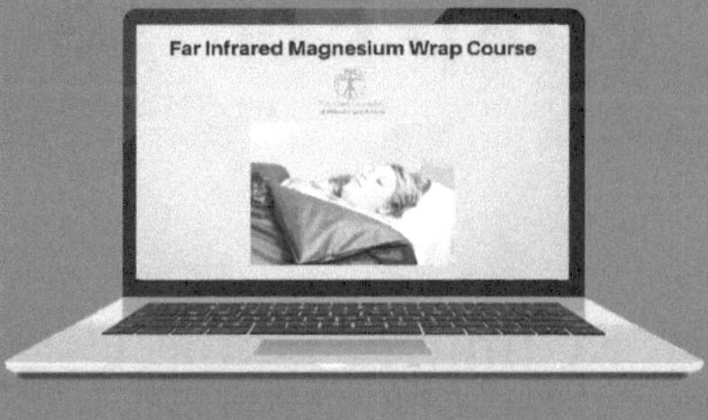

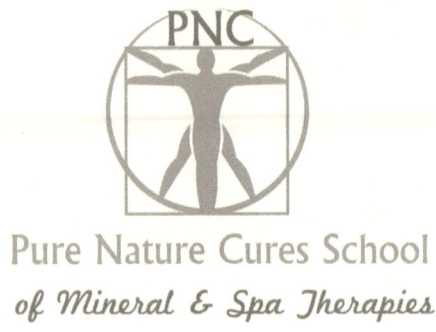

Far Infrared Magnesium Wrap Course

for Clinic & Home Use

Galina St George

Far Infrared Magnesium Wrap Course - Galina St George

All Rights Reserved. No part of this publication may be reproduced in any form or by any means, including scanning, photocopying, or otherwise without prior written permission of the copyright holder.
Copyright © 2021

Far Infrared Magnesium Wrap Course - Galina St George

Table of Contents

Introduction..7
Disclaimer..12
Module 1 - Course Overview: Resources, Certification, Materials and Equipment, Disclaimer and Therapist Qualification Requirements..14
    Unit 1 - Course Overview: Resources, Certification and Other Details..14
    Unit 2 – Disclaimer..17
    Unit 3 - Therapist Qualification Requirements..................23
Module 2 - The Skin - Its Structure and Functions. The Role of Skin in Mineral Supplementation and Pain Management...........26
    Unit 1 - The Skin - Its Structure and Functions..................26
        There are 6 skin functions:..................................32
    Unit 2 – The Role of the Skin in Mineral Supplementation and Pain Management..34
Module 3 - Anatomy of a Nerve Cell. Types of Pain. Magnesium for Muscle Cramps. Managing Pain with Magnesium................38
    Unit 1 - Anatomy of a Nerve Cell. Types of Pain..................38
    Unit 2 - Magnesium for Muscle Cramps..........................43
    Unit 3 - Managing Pain with Magnesium..........................46
Module 4 - Link Between Pain and Inflammation. Acute vs Chronic Inflammation. How Inflammation Affects Our Health..49
    Unit 1 - Link Between Pain and Inflammation.....................49
    Unit 2 - Acute vs Chronic Inflammation..........................52
    Unit 3 - How Inflammation Affects Our Health...................54
Module 5 - Pain and Inflammation Management Methods Used in Allopathic Medicine. Their Side-effects..................................58
    Unit 1 - Pain and Inflammation Management Methods Used in Allopathic Medicine. Side-Effects..................................58
        NSAIDs..60
        COX-2 inhibitors..60
            Steroids..61
            Medical marijuana..62
            Opioids..63

Conclusion..64
Module 6 - Far Infrared Rays - How They Work. Therapeutic Benefits & Uses..65
    Unit 1 - Far Infrared Energy - How It Works. How FIR Interacts with the Body..65
    Unit 2 - Therapeutic Benefits and Uses of Far Infrared..........71
Module 7 - Importance of Magnesium for Health. What Causes Magnesium Deficiency, and Why It Is Dangerous to Health.......78
    Unit 1 - Importance of Magnesium for Health........................78
    Unit 2 - What Causes Magnesium Deficiency, and Why It Is Dangerous to Health...83
Module 8 - Magnesium Supplementation Methods. Transdermal vs Oral Supplementation - Advantages and Disadvantages..........92
    Unit 1 - Magnesium Supplementation Methods......................92
    Unit 2 - Transdermal vs Oral Supplementation......................94
Module 9 - Products and Methods Used in Transdermal Magnesium Supplementation. Magnesium Chloride vs Magnesium Sulphate..97
    Unit 1 - Products and Methods Used in Transdermal Magnesium Supplementation..97
    Unit 2 - Magnesium Chloride vs Magnesium Sulphate.......100
Module 10 - Managing Pain Using Far Infrared and Magnesium 105
    Unit 1 - Managing Pain Using Far Infrared..........................105
    Unit 2 - Managing Pain Using Magnesium..........................108
Module 11 - Far Infrared Magnesium Pain and Health Management Wrap..112
    Unit 1 - FIR Magnesium Pain and Health Management Wrap - Benefits, Uses, Contraindications, Cautions..........................112
    Unit 2 - Products, Materials and Equipment........................126
    Unit 3 - Far Infrared Magnesium Wrap Procedure...............129
Module 12 - Other Conditions Far Infrared Magnesium Wrap Can Help With..139
    Unit 1 - Other Conditions Far Infrared Magnesium Wrap Can Help With..139
Module 13 - Case studies and Practical Training......................143

Far Infrared Magnesium Wrap Course - Galina St George

    Unit 1 – Case Studies...143
    Unit 2 - Consultation Form..145
    Unit 3 - Practical Training..146
Further Information..148
    Mineral Healing Books...148
    Courses..149

Introduction

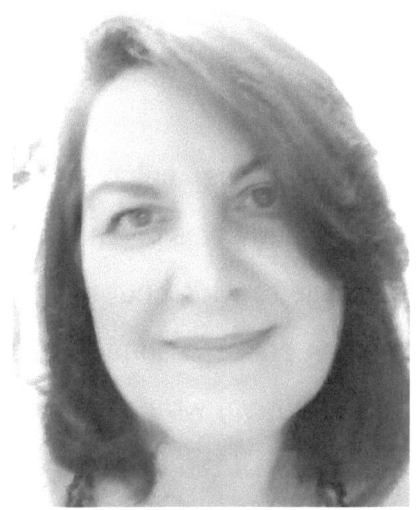

Far Infrared Magnesium Wrap was the first treatment I decided to create a course for when I realised how powerful transdermal magnesium applications were when they were combined with the far-infrared technology.

I did the first treatment on a Yoga instructor called Joe, in the middle of a cold and rainy December day. She came a long way and was stressed because of a long drive. She was also shivering with cold. Luckily, the blanket had already been warmed up, so the first thing she did was to take a long deep sigh of relief and sheer pleasure. Imagine yourself being cold, stressed and tired being put on a soft warm bed! I think we can all relate to the pleasure it brings.

However, this was only the beginning of 2-hour pampering experience. Joe's tired body was given an hour-long magnesium oil massage to which put her to sleep halfway through. She was then put on a sheet soaked in magnesium chloride solution, wrapped up in it and covered with the top part of the far-infrared blanket. In her own words, it felt like being wrapped in a warm cocoon.

Here is what she wrote: "Imagine yourself being scrubbed and massaged gently but deeply – to ease your aches and pains, then being placed in a warm cocoon for an hour or so. You are deeply relaxed, your mind is so relaxed that you are falling asleep. You are feeling so wonderful that you want it to last and last..."

Joe said to me that it was just what she needed. Being a Yoga instructor can be tough on the muscles and joints.

To add to that, she had a hard time with her business, so was feeling very stressed. The treatment addressed both her mental and physical problems by bringing profound relaxation and a feeling of pure bliss.

Apart from the psychological benefits of being cared for, her body was warmed through on a very deep level with far infrared which also helped to speed up the delivery of magnesium ions to all the body cells.

Magnesium is the 4th most abundant element in the body. We need it for over 300 body processes. It takes part in the formation of neurotransmitters, hormones, muscle and bone tissues. It takes care of the normal muscle and nerve function, steady heart rhythm, normal blood pressure, healthy immune system and strong bones. It also helps to maintain blood sugar at normal levels. It plays a vital role in preventing heart disease, diabetes, cancer, osteoporosis and a whole range of other issues.

Among other things, magnesium deficiency in many people has led to a rise in obesity, diabetes, chronic fatigue, depression, anxiety, heart attacks, cancer and many other physical and mental problems.

The big issue with magnesium is that while food is seen as the best way to keep its levels stable, our food has become poor in magnesium due to the soil growing food becoming impoverished due to extensive agriculture methods. I have read many research pieces which show how magnesium-poor soil contributes to a rise in heart disease and cancer.

What can we do? Many of us take magnesium supplements. However, not everybody can benefit from oral supplementation. First of all, as we age, our intestinal tract becomes clogged with all sorts of mucus which makes absorption of nutrients much less effective, so much of oral magnesium just passes through the body. Second, you need to take it for a substantial time to reduce an imbalance. Third, there is always a risk of taking too much which at best can cause diarrhoea and at worst affect the kidneys, especially in people with kidney problems.

This makes a very good case for transdermal supplementation. The skin is a wonderful organ which can regulate what comes into the body and how much. Far Infrared Magnesium Wraps are a very fast way to reduce magnesium deficiency bringing a whole range of benefits with it.

Moreover, far infrared technology is in itself very powerful – in promoting magnesium ion absorption, softening the tissues and facilitating sweating which helps to remove toxic waste. You can read about all the other benefits of magnesium salts and far-infrared when you go through the course modules.

The course is aimed both at therapists and members of the public who want to help improve their health. I hope that having read the book you will decide to enrol on the online course and get certified to offer the treatment to your clients. Please get in touch with me regarding enrolment details and any questions you might have.

Galina St George

Disclaimer

The author of this material sincerely believes that a natural approach to health and maintaining a natural balance within the human body are very important in experiencing energy, vitality, and vibrant health throughout life.

The author recognizes that opinions within scientific and medical fields differ greatly. The purpose of this book is to share educational information and scientific research gathered by the author, scientists, and informed advocates of health and wellbeing using natural methods and resources.

None of the information contained in this book is intended to diagnose, prevent, treat, or cure any disease, nor is it intended to prescribe any of the techniques, materials or concepts presented as a form of treatment for any illness or medical condition. Before beginning any practice regarding the procedures described in the book, it is highly recommended that you first obtain the consent and advice of licensed health care professional.

The information given in this book should be used for educational purposes only, and not as advice or prescription for specific medical conditions. Responsibility for any action taken as a result of reading this book will lie solely with you. The author assumes no responsibility for the choices you make after you review the information contained herein and your consultation with a licensed healthcare professional.

If you are on medication, do not start taking or using minerals without consulting with your GP since minerals can interfere with medicines.

Module 1 - Course Overview: Resources, Certification, Materials and Equipment, Disclaimer and Therapist Qualification Requirements.

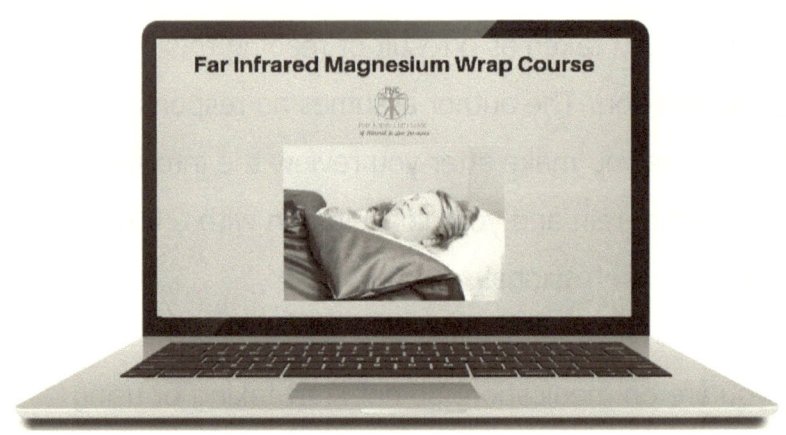

Unit 1 - Course Overview: Resources, Certification and Other Details

Course Overview

Far Infrared Magnesium Wrap Course is one of a range of courses developed by Pure Nature Cures School of Mineral & Spa Therapies. The course explores multiple health benefits of magnesium and various transdermal applications of magnesium salts.

Who Is This Course Suitable For?

1. Therapists with a valid Level 3 Anatomy & Physiology + Massage qualifications - to obtain professional insurance and be able to practice professionally.
2. Members of the public who would like to learn the course for their own needs.

Resources

1. Course units
2. Recommended literature & websites.

Certification

The course has been approved by the International Institute of Holistic Therapists. Certification is issued by the Pure Nature Cures School of Mineral & Spa Therapies.

To get certified, you will need to go through our online course and complete the test questions after corresponding units.

Everyone who has completed the course units and quizzes will be issued with a certificate of completion.

If you decide to qualify as a therapist, you will need to complete an add-on unit for therapists, case studies, the practical module and assignments. This will qualify you for the practitioner certificate which you can use to apply for professional insurance.

You will need to make enquiries with your local insurance providers to obtain professional insurance.

Materials & Equipment Needed for the Treatment

1. Magnesium oil, magnesium salts (essential)
2. Far infrared blanket
3. Other components which will be described later in the course.

Unit 2 – Disclaimer

Medical Disclaimer

Neither I personally nor my business makes any representations or guarantees in terms of medical information and research materials described in this Course, express or implied. All information in this Course is presented solely for educational purposes, and not to diagnose or treat any person for any medical symptom, illness or condition.

None of the information, treatments and techniques presented in this Course, in written or oral communication, within our Practical modules, webinars and consultations is meant to replace or teach to replace medical diagnosis or treatment. Students are always encouraged to seek medical diagnosis and treatment for any medical problems.

While we aim to present what we believe to be complete, accurate and true information, considering a diversity of views in the medical research field, we cannot guarantee that the information in this Course is always complete, accurate and true. This does exempt us from any liabilities and responsibilities which may not be excluded by applicable legislation.

It is a responsibility of the Reader/ Student/ Therapist to assess their own or their client's health and to make an appropriate decision regarding the suitability of advice or treatment in each particular case. Written consent of the 3rd party must always be obtained before any advice or treatment is provided.

We list some contra-indications to the treatments described in our course materials. However, the list is not exhaustive. The Reader/ Student/ Therapist must always make their assessment of any conditions the 3rd party presents them with and decide whether a treatment is appropriate for themselves or their client.

We will not be held responsible for 3rd party decisions, consultations, treatments or results of these which happen outside the premises and the schedule of the Practical Module Course.

Professional Advice Disclaimer

Neither the information contained within this Course nor communication between the Course Provider/ Book Author/ Business on one hand and Reader/ Student/ Therapist on the other hand, in any form or on any subject – such as medicine, pharmacology, psychology, finances, commerce, marketing, taxes, accounting, must be regarded nor used as a substitution for professional advice.

Earnings Disclaimer

Neither the information on this Website nor digital or other forms of communication between the Reader/ Student/ Therapist are meant to offer any guarantees in terms of potential earnings.

You accept that financial and another type of success depend on a variety of factors, such as knowledge, skills, abilities, dedication, experience, strategies, marketing efforts, networking, the spending power of your potential clients, etc.

As a professional therapist, you are the only person responsible for your earnings and financial success. While we outline revenue potential as a result of the skills you have learned with us, we cannot give any promises or guarantees in this respect, and no statements on this website aim to mislead you in this respect.

Persons under 16

Persons under 16 years of age require their parent's permission to use materials, treatments and techniques, as well as to receive a consultation or a treatment described in this Course. It is the responsibility of a Reader/ Student/ Therapist to ensure that such permission has been obtained before a consultation or a treatment has been provided to a person who is under 16 years of age.

Personal & Professional Responsibility

Far Infrared Magnesium Wrap Course - Galina St George

You agree that you are solely responsible for your own professional (public, product and any other relevant type) liability as a result of your actions. You are the only person responsible for your compliance with the law and regulations in any area of your business.

You agree that by using this Course information and Services, you take full responsibility for your own decisions, actions and results of your actions towards yourself or 3rd parties. You agree to comply with laws and legislation of the country you live in. You are solely responsible for your Professional Indemnity Insurance, National Insurance and taxes.

We highly recommend that you make enquiries about membership of professional organisations and professional liability insurance before you start treating clients. You should always work in the interests of your clients (paying or non-paying) and within the framework of legal and ethical considerations.

Far Infrared Magnesium Wrap Course - Galina St George

All the courses and treatments presented by Pure Nature Cures School of Mineral & Spa Therapies are being marketed as complementary health and beauty courses and treatments, and are not meant to promote or endorse any medical information, or provide diagnosis and/or medical treatment.

Contraindications to Treatments

If you have any medical condition, please address it with a medical professional. The treatments have certain contra-indications, so are not suitable for everyone. See the **list of common contra-indications here.**

There may be other conditions not listed here which may make a person unsuitable for treatment. If you are unsure, please refer your client to a medical professional. Never conduct treatment without consultation to establish a client's suitability for the procedure.

Pure Nature Cures School of Mineral & Spa Therapies offers no diagnosis or treatment of problems of a medical nature, and no guarantees in terms of health benefits described within the Course.

While there are multiple possible benefits to the treatments, they should be seen as part of the integrative approach to health issues rather than a sole option. Any positive results will depend on a combination of factors taken by you or your client, and we cannot and do not offer any guarantees in terms of benefits mentioned within our offers or the course syllabus.

Please let us know if you have any questions, and we will be happy to reply. You can contact us by email: **support@purenaturecures.com**.

For more detailed information about the terms and conditions of using our website and training please see **Terms**.

Unit 3 - Therapist Qualification Requirements

Far Infrared Magnesium Wrap Course - Galina St George

The courses run by the Pure Nature Cures School of Mineral & Spa Therapies are aimed both at therapists and members of the public.

1. Members of the public take our courses to learn about the health benefits of salts, clays and minerals and do treatments on themselves, based on their assessment of their health. In the case of existing health issues, members of the public should always seek medical advice before having a treatment. Even though the majority of people will benefit from the treatments, some people may find them unsuitable. **Read about some of the contra-indications and cautions here.**

2. Our courses can also be taken by qualified therapists who would like to add new skills to their portfolio. To be considered qualified, a therapist needs to have a Level 3 Anatomy & Physiology and Body Massage Diploma.

3. While all the students will be issued with the Certificate of Completion, only qualified therapists will receive a Practitioner Certificate which will allow them to

apply for Practitioner insurance and treat members of the public.

4. We cannot guarantee that the qualification we offer will be accepted by insurers in the country of your residence, due to variations regarding requirements for complementary therapies. Please make enquiries with your local insurance providers.

5. To qualify as a therapist, you will need to sign up for the add-on short course for therapists which covers subjects such as hygiene, professional issues, as well as case studies.

6. The optional practical one-day module is offered to therapists in the UK & Northern Ireland, as well as to those who can travel to the UK for the course.

Module 2 - The Skin - Its Structure and Functions. The Role of Skin in Mineral Supplementation and Pain Management.

Unit 1 - The Skin - Its Structure and Functions

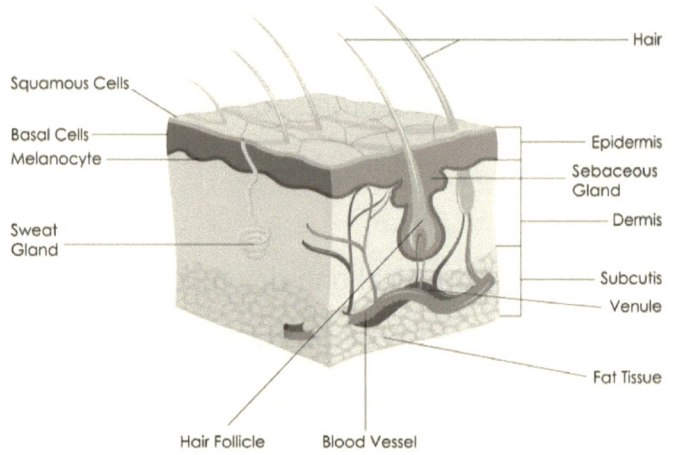

Skin Structure

Skin is a remarkable organ of the body which can perform various vital functions. It can mould to different shapes, stretch and harden, but can also feel a delicate touch, pain, pressure, hot and cold, and is an effective communicator between the outside environment and the brain.

The skin makes up to 12-15% of an adult's body weight. Each square centimetre has 6 million cells, 5,000 sensory points, 100 sweat glands and 15 sebaceous glands. It consists of 3 layers: the epidermis (the outer layer), the dermis ('true skin') and the subcutaneous (fat) layer.

Skin is constantly being regenerated. A skin cell starts its life at the lower layer of the skin (the basal layer of the dermis), which is supplied with blood vessels and nerve ending. The cell migrates upward for about two weeks until it reaches the bottom portion of the epidermis, which is the outermost skin layer.

The epidermis is not supplied with blood vessels but has nerve endings. For another 2 weeks, the cell undergoes a series of changes in the epidermis, gradually flattening out and moving toward the surface. Then it dies and is shed. Below is a detailed diagram of the skin structure.

Epidermis

The main function of the epidermis is to form a tough barrier against between the body and the outside world, while the dermis is a soft, thick cushion of connective tissue that lies directly below the epidermis and largely determines the way our skin looks. Both layers keep repairing and renewing themselves throughout or life, but the dermis does it more slowly than the epidermis.

Under the dermis is a layer of fat cells, which is known as adipose tissue (or subcutaneous fat layer). It provides insulation and protective padding for the body. It also provides an emergency energy supply.

The epidermis consists of 5 layers:

1. Basal layer (Stratum germinativum) - this is the bottom layer of the skin. The cells of this layer constantly been reproduced, since they contain a nucleus or seed. As the cells reproduce, the layers get constantly pushed up into the next layer.

2. Prickle cell layer (Stratum spinosum) - called this way because the cells have spines which prevent bacteria from entering the cells and moisture being lost. These cells also have a nucleus and therefore reproduce.

3. Granular layer (Stratum granulosum) - the prickle cells lose their spines and become flattered. The nucleus dies, and protein is formed called keratin. This protein prevents moisture loss and is found in skin, nails and hair.

4. Clear layer (Stratum lucidum) - this layer is for cushioning and protection and is found only on the palms of the hands and soles of the feet.

5. Horny (cornified) layer (Stratum corneum) - the cells here are dead and ready to be shed (desquamation). This process speeds up as we age.

Dermis

The dermis is the layer responsible for the skin's structural integrity, elasticity and resilience. Wrinkles develop in the dermis. Therefore, an anti-wrinkle treatment has a chance to succeed only if it can reach the dermis. Typical collagen and elastin creams, for example, never reach the dermis because collagen and elastin molecules are too large to penetrate the epidermis. Hence, contrary to what some manufacturers of such creams might claim, these creams have little effect on skin wrinkles.

The dermis is the middle layer of the skin located between the epidermis and subcutaneous tissue. It is the thickest of the skin layers and comprises a tight, sturdy mesh of collagen and elastin fibres. Both collagen and elastin are critically important skin proteins: collagen is responsible for the structural support and elastin for the resilience of the skin.

The key type of cells in the dermis is fibroblasts, which synthesize collagen, elastin and other structural molecules. The proper function of fibroblasts is highly important for overall skin health. The dermis also contains capillaries (tiny blood vessels) and lymph nodes which produce immune cells. Blood capillaries are responsible for bringing oxygen and nutrients to the skin and removing carbon dioxide and products of cell metabolism (what we call waste matter).

Lymph nodes are engaged in protecting the skin from invading microorganisms.

Finally, the dermis contains sebaceous glands, sweat glands, hair follicles and a small number of nerve and muscle cells. Sebaceous glands, based around hair follicles, produce sebum, an oily protective substance that lubricates the skin and hair and provides protection by forming an acid mantle when mixed with sweat. When a sebaceous gland produces too little sebum which is common in older people, the skin becomes excessively dry and more prone to wrinkling. Too much of sebum, as is common in teenagers, often leads to acne.

The dermis is thicker than the epidermis but has fewer cells. It consists mainly of connective tissue which is made up of fibres of the proteins collagen and elastin and a non-fibrous gelatin-like material called ground substance or extracellular matrix.

Subcutaneous tissue

Subcutaneous tissue is the deepest layer of the skin located under the dermis and consisting mainly of fat cells. It acts as a shock absorber and heat insulator, protecting underlying tissues from cold and trauma. The loss of subcutaneous tissue in later years leads to facial sag and makes wrinkles more visible. To counteract it, a cosmetic procedure where fat is taken from elsewhere in the body and injected into facial areas is common these days.

Skin Functions

There are 6 skin functions:

Sensation - the nerve endings in the skin identify touch, heat, cold, pain and light pressure.

Heat regulation - the skin helps to regulate the body temperature by sweating to cool the body down when it overheats and shivering creating 'goose bumps' when it is cold. Shivering closes the pores. The tiny hair that stands on end traps warm air and thus helps keep the body warm.

Absorption - absorption of ultraviolet rays from the sun helps to form vitamin D in the body, which is vital for bone formation. Some creams, essential oils and medicines (e.g. HRT, anti-smoking patches) can also be absorbed through the skin into the bloodstream.

Protection - the skin protects the body from ultraviolet light - too much of it is harmful to the body - by producing a pigment called melanin. It also protects us from the invasion of bacteria and germs by forming an acid mantle (formed by the skin sebum and sweat). This barrier also prevents moisture loss.

Excretion - Waste products and toxins are eliminated from the body through the sweat glands. It is a very important function which helps to keep the body 'clean' from the inside.

Secretion - sebum and sweat are secreted onto the skin surface. The sebum keeps the skin lubricated and soft, and the sweat combines with the sebum to form an acid mantle which creates the right pH balance for the skin to fight off infection.

I would add **one more very important** but frequently overlooked **function** to this list: **diagnostic**. The skin shows the state of our health. So, when we are ill or otherwise unhealthy, the skin will reflect it immediately. Toxic, congested, tired, stressed body will often have pale, unhealthy complexion. Deprived of proper nourishment and good oxygen supply due to inefficient circulation and elimination, it will be more prone to various skin problems.

Further Reading

1. Skin Structure & Function. http://www.merckmanuals.com/home/skin_disorders/biology_of_the_skin/structure_and_function_of_the_skin.html
2. Skin Structure & Function. http://courses.washington.edu/bioen327/Labs/Lit_SkinStruct_Bensouillah_Ch01.pdf

Unit 2 – The Role of the Skin in Mineral Supplementation and Pain Management

Transdermal therapies rely on **2 main functions** of the skin to work:

1. **Absorption**
2. **Excretion**

Both functions are possible due to the permeability of the skin thanks to its microporous structure. A large number of pores allows the skin to absorb various salts. aroma oils and even larger organic molecules of medicines. This function is very important in terms of transdermal mineral supplementation.

The same pores also allow the skin to release toxins. Excretion is a process opposite to absorption, with the skin releasing unwanted substances and water out of the body. Without this ability, the body systems would fail very quickly, because the body systems will not be able to take the pressure. The skin takes upon itself a very important function to rid the body of toxins bypassing other channels, such as the liver and kidneys. This is why in cases of severe skin damage (due to burns for example), the body systems can fail very quickly - especially the kidneys.

The skin is very large if laid out and stretched, which allows it to work very efficiently. Of course, the skin by itself would be nothing without the network of multiple capillaries take away toxins to the skin surface for elimination. The same network delivers important nutrients from the surface of the skin to the cells inside the body. Salt ions are easiest for the skin to absorb and excrete, due to their minute size. They come out with sweat and get inside the body when it is sprayed, massaged or submerged in a salty solution.

And here we should mention another remarkable property of the skin - called **"osmosis"**. No matter how salty the water is (e.g. Dead Sea water is over-saturated with salt), the skin will not take more salt than necessary (unlike when salt is taken orally). The skin regulates the intake of salts in a very intelligent way, stopping any salt overload. This means that salt-water balance is maintained at all times if one relies on supplementing minerals transdermally, as opposed to oral supplementation. No matter how salty the water in the sea, we do not become "overdosed" with salt from swimming in it.

Thanks to these properties of the skin, transdermal magnesium therapy is a very safe way to supplement magnesium which when in the body starts interacting with the Central and Peripheral Nervous systems to help reduce and manage pain in various parts of the body. Magnesium also helps to reduce inflammation which in turn leads to a reduction in painful symptoms. Oral supplementation works in a much slower way and is not always efficient. This brings us to the conclusion that the skin plays a vital role in reducing and managing pain and inflammation.

Further Reading

1. 6 Ways to Detox through Your Skin. http://www.mindbodygreen.com/0-1683/6-Ways-to-Detox-Through-Your-Skin.html
2. Arsenic, Cadmium, Lead, and Mercury in Sweat: A Systematic Review. Margaret E. Sears et al. http://www.hindawi.com/journals/jeph/2012/184745/
3. Mineral Supplements May Be Used Via the Skin. http://www.naturalnews.com/010061_minerals_skin_supplements.html

Module 3 - Anatomy of a Nerve Cell. Types of Pain. Magnesium for Muscle Cramps. Managing Pain with Magnesium.

Unit 1 - Anatomy of a Nerve Cell. Types of Pain.

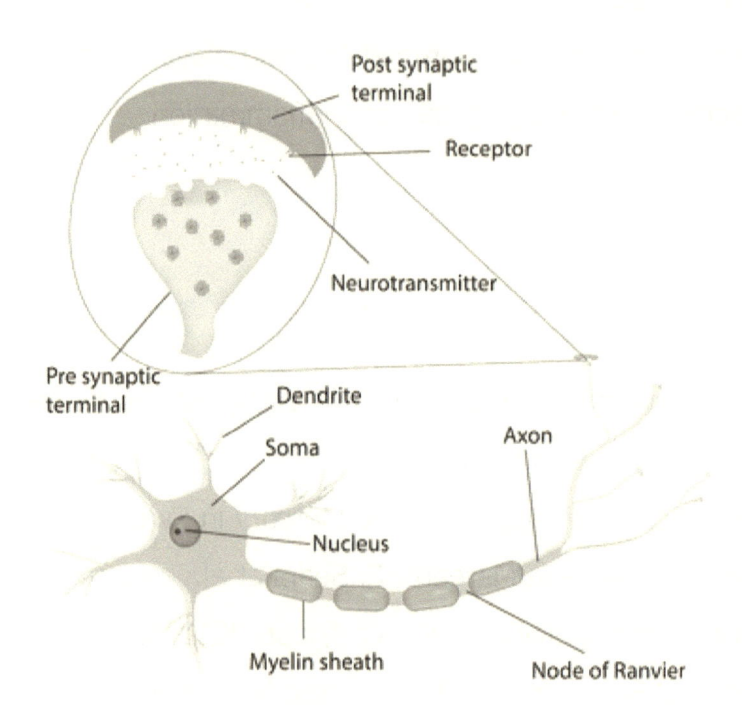

Anatomy of a Nerve Cell

Pain is a signal that something is not right. Its main goal is to protect the body from harm. The nervous system can normally tell the difference between the pain signals which may be harmful and those which are not, instinctively, by-passing the cognitive part of the brain.

The nervous system consists of two major parts:

1. The central nervous system which includes the brain and the spinal cord
2. The peripheral nervous system comprising all the other nerves.

The main building block of the nervous system is a **nerve cell or neuron**. It consists of:

1. Cell body (soma) - the main part of a neuron where the nucleus is found.
2. Dendrites - projections radiating from the neuron in all directions. A single neuron can have up to 200 of them. They receive signals to the nerve.

3. Axon, which is sometimes covered with myelin sheath - the fatty coating which protects the axon and speeds up nerve signal transmission.
4. Synaptic end bulb - the swelling at the end of the nerve cell which contains the neurotransmitter.
5. Synapse - a space which separates the end bulb from an adjacent nerve cell or dendrite.
6. The node of Ranvier - a gap in the myelin sheath which helps the conduction of the nerve impulse.

"Nerve impulses travel along neurons in the form of electrical signals. These signals cross the synapses (tiny gaps) between one neuron and the next in the chemical form before being transmitted again in electrical form. Signals are also chemically transmitted to other target cells, such as those in muscles, which make appropriate responses." **Source**

Pain and response to it are transmitted to and from the brain via nerve cells. Types of nerves include sensory and motor nerves. Sensory nerves carry messages from the body to the brain. The response is carried from the brain to the body by the motor nerves. It is the sensory nerves that trigger the reflex that pulls us away from pain.

Most sensory and motor nerves are enclosed in a myelin sheath that acts as a conductor for impulses in the nerve fibre. The signals between neurons are electric by nature and are transmitted from one cell to other thanks to neurotransmitters, and there is a range of these in the body.

Types & Causes of Pain

Somatic Pain - sharp and localised. It is felt in the skin, muscles, joints and ligaments. The nerve receptors with this type of pain are sensitive to pressure, temperature, stretch, vibration. They are also sensitive to inflammation, as would happen if you cut yourself, sprain something that causes tissue damage. It also includes pain as a result of lack of oxygen, as in ischemic muscle cramps.

Visceral Pain is felt in the internal organs and main body cavities - the thorax (lungs and heart), abdomen (bowel, spleen, liver and kidneys), and the pelvis (ovaries, bladder, and the womb). The pain receptors sense inflammation, stretch and ischemia (oxygen starvation). Visceral pain is harder to localise, and the sensation is more like a deep dull ache. This is why pain is often referred to as "ache". It can also radiate to other body organs.

Nerve Pain (Neuropathic Pain) comes from within the nervous system itself. You may have heard people referring to a pinched or trapped nerve. The pain can originate from the nerves between the tissues and the spinal cord (peripheral nervous system) and the nerves between the spinal cord and the brain (central nervous system). It can be caused by nerve degeneration, for example as a result of a stroke or oxygen starvation. It may also be due to a trapped nerve, which puts pressure on it. Nerve infection in the case of shingles or a torn/slipped intervertebral disc can cause this kind of pain.

Sympathetic Pain The sympathetic nervous system controls the blood flow to our skin and muscles, perspiration, and the speed of functioning of the peripheral nervous system. Sympathetic pain happens after a fracture or a soft tissue injury of the limbs. There are no specific pain receptors with this type of pain. As with neuropathic pain, the nerve is injured, becomes unstable and fires off random, abnormal signals to the brain, which interprets them as pain. With this type of pain, the skin and the area around the injury become extremely sensitive. The pain can virtually immobilise a limb, which if lasting too long can cause other problems, such as muscle wasting, osteoporosis, arthritis, and joint stiffness.

Unit 2 - Magnesium for Muscle Cramps

Cramps of any kind are sudden, involuntary contractions of muscles or muscles. Most common cramps are experienced in the calf muscles and the soles of the feet and occur during the night or while at rest.

Cramps can also affect other muscles in the body in people of any age group. Stomach cramps are quite common, especially with women of reproductive age.

There may be various causes for cramps to happen. Scientific research has not identified a precise reason for muscle cramps. However, it may be due to the nerves controlling the muscles rather than the muscles themselves.

Leg cramps can be caused by over-exertion of the muscles, structural disorders (such as flat feet), prolonged sitting, standing on a hard surface, or dehydration. Less common causes include diabetes, hypoglycemia, anaemia, thyroid and endocrine dysfunction, Parkinson's and certain medications.

Low levels of certain minerals acting as electrolytes in the body - they include magnesium, potassium, sodium and calcium - have long been linked to leg cramps. It especially affects long-distance runners and cyclists. Diuretics can also cause leg cramps. Pregnant women are also more susceptible to leg cramps.

"Canadian doctors have found that magnesium supplements can alleviate muscle cramps. In severe cases, magnesium has been provided intravenously and this has led to the relief of symptoms within 24 hours. Many cases of muscle cramps are caused by low concentrations of magnesium in the blood... The reason why it helps is due to diuretic medications or strenuous exercise. When taken orally, it seems that magnesium glucoheptonate or magnesium gluconate works best". Bilbey, Douglas L, Prabhakaran V.M. Muscle cramps and magnesium deficiency: case reports. Canadian Family Physician. July http://www.internethealthlibrary.com/Health-problems/Muscle%20cramps%20-%20researchDiet&Lifestyle.htm

Dr John Briffa says: "I remember once attending a nutritional therapy course for doctors in the US, in which one of the facilitators (Dr Jonathan Wright) said, "If it spasms, think magnesium" (or something similar). And this sage piece of advice was based on the idea that low levels of magnesium in the body tend to cause a muscle to go into spasm. This might include so-called 'smooth' muscle in, say, the digestive tract, bladder on in the walls of the arteries. It might also include 'skeletal' muscle, say, in the legs. Ever since hearing learning this, I've used magnesium generally very effectively to treat conditions like muscular cramps, 'restless legs', irritable bladder syndrome and oesophageal spasm".

To prevent cramps from happening, magnesium, potassium and sodium levels have to be monitored - especially in people who lose a lot of fluids due to exercise, excessive sweating, vomiting or diarrhoea. Magnesium is best absorbed by the body when applied transdermally. It is the quickest method too.

Unit 3 - Managing Pain with Magnesium

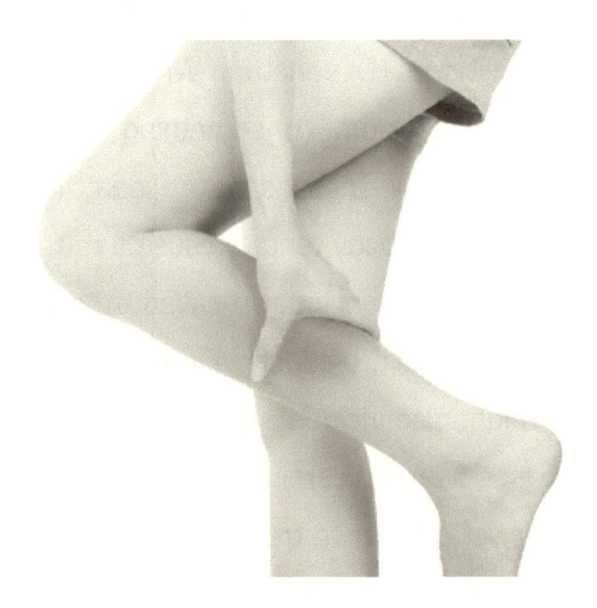

Magnesium is one of the most powerful natural relaxants in nature. It also has a profound effect on the functioning of the nervous system. Without sufficient magnesium, nerves start firing signals too easily with even a minor stimulus. Noises become too loud, lights too bright, emotions exaggerated. Magnesium is known to regulate or inhibit many nerve receptors. It acts like water on fire cooling down the nervous system.

Magnesium also appears to be able to affect the nervous system by regulating the release of hormones, which occurs due to many different forms of stress. "Without enough magnesium, serotonin flows unchecked, constricting blood vessels and releasing other pain-producing chemicals such as substance P and prostaglandins, he says. Normal magnesium levels not only prevent the release of these pain-producing substances but also stop their effects, says Dr Altura." http://www.mgwater.com/prev1801.shtml

Unfortunately, it is very difficult to determine magnesium deficiency using a blood test, since blood serum level does not reflect the amount of magnesium in the tissues. This is the reason it often gets overlooked, and unnoticed, with dire consequences to health. Also, it is difficult to achieve optimal magnesium levels via oral supplementation.

The reason for it is that magnesium is not easily absorbed by the digestive system. If digestion is compromised due to an IBS, gluten intolerance, or leaky gut, then supplementation becomes an even greater challenge. To add to it a diet high in processed foods which contain phosphates, and much oral magnesium will pass through the body unabsorbed.

Further Reading

1. Inflammation & Pain Management with Magnesium. http://drsircus.com/medicine/magnesium/inflammation-and-systemic-stress
2. Magnesium Treats Fibromyalgia Pain. http://www.fmnetnews.com/latest-news/magnesium-treats-fibromyalgia-pain

Module 4 - Link Between Pain and Inflammation. Acute vs Chronic Inflammation. How Inflammation Affects Our Health.

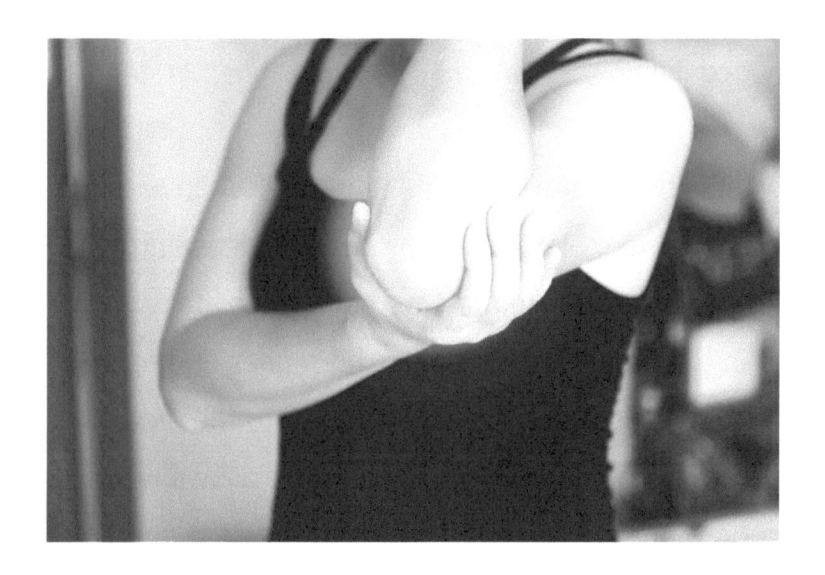

Unit 1 - Link Between Pain and Inflammation

Inflammation is the body's immune response to damage caused to itself. The body makes an effort to heal itself after an injury defending itself against viruses and bacteria. It is also a focused effort to repair damaged tissues.

Without this response, the damage would get worse and infections would deteriorate and become deadly. However, inflammation can also cause a lot of problems when it becomes chronic. Inflammation is often accompanied by redness, heat, swelling, pain and inability to move the damaged limb.

So what is the anatomy of inflammation? When we dislocate a knee, biochemical processes release proteins called cytokines. These are emergency mediators which bring in the body's immune cells, hormones and nutrients to fix the problem. Blood flow increases to the area, capillaries become more permeable. This allows white blood cells, hormones and nutrients to move into the spaces between cells.

White blood cells called leukocytes and phagocytes swarm the injured area and ingest germs, dead or damaged cells and other foreign materials to help heal the body. Then we have hormones called prostaglandins to create blood clots. This is done to help heal the damaged tissues and remove them when healing is finished.

The process is accompanied by what is called "nociceptive pain" - a type of pain which is often a result of an injury. It usually goes away when the damaged part heals. The tissue damage caused by inflammation results in a chain of biochemical responses which provoke the nervous system to respond by sending pain signals to the brain.

Long-term inflammation can cause adaptive responses in the nervous system which results in exaggerated pain and tenderness in and around the damaged tissues - often referred to as "neuropathic (or nerve) pain".

In cases of chronic inflammation the number of cytokines, white blood cells and hormones in the inflamed tissues increases which means that pain becomes worse. For this reason, reducing inflammation would lead to a reduction in pain sensations.

Inflammation is normally caused by tissue damage. This results in a chain of biochemical responses which provoke the nervous system to respond by sending pain signals to the brain. Long-term inflammation can cause adaptive responses in the nervous system which results in exaggerated pain and tenderness in and around the damaged tissues.

Allopathic medicine uses anti-inflammatory non-steroid (NSAIDs) and steroid-based drugs to deal with inflammation. As we will see in one of the following modules, such drugs have often very serious side effects.

This creates a need to look for natural alternatives where possible, and magnesium salts present a great alternative due to their anti-inflammatory properties.

Unit 2 - Acute vs Chronic Inflammation

Like with the types of pain, there are two types of inflammation - **acute** and **chronic**.

Acute inflammation happens just after an injury. Its purpose is to ensure a speedy recovery. In cases of acute inflammation, the area becomes painful, red and swollen, sometimes hot. This type of inflammation is fast developing and doesn't last long.

Examples of acute inflammation are a *scraped elbow, stubbed toe, sprained ankle, dislocated joint, tooth abscess, earache, cystitis, sciatica, sty or boil*. All of these invoke a powerful body response resulting in inflammation.

Normally acute inflammation doesn't last long. It goes away when an affected area has been through a process of healing.

Chronic inflammation lasts over a long time. Examples of chronic inflammation are *osteoarthritis, rheumatism, Crohn's disease, gingivitis, allergies, asthma, gout, heart disease* and more. Factors like stress, *environmental pollution, poor diet, lack of exercise, excess weight* contribute to the length and severity of chronic inflammation, often being the primary cause of it in the first place.

Chronic inflammation is considered low-grade, progressing slowly and often goes unnoticed. However, it doesn't make it less dangerous. Chronic inflammation is more deadly than acute since it is often ignored until too late. The test which is an indicator of the presence of chronic inflammation is a test for the c-reactive protein (CRP) which is elevated in such cases.

Unit 3 - How Inflammation Affects Our Health

While acute inflammation normally progresses rather fast and unless one is very unlucky, heals fast too, it is chronic inflammation that often leads to long-term complications and chronic (even life-threatening) conditions which include:

- Diabetes
- Heart disease
- Bone & joint problems
- Depression
- Aggressive behaviour
- Respiratory conditions
- Skin problems
- Cancer.

Diabetes - scientific research has established that chronic inflammation can result in cytokines interfering with insulin signalling which results in insulin resistance and elevated blood sugar levels. This leads to white blood cells attacking healthy tissues which leads to worsening of inflammation.

Heart disease - chronic inflammation leads to the deposition of cholesterol in the blood vessel lining. They cytokines attack the deposits which in turn leads to worsening of inflammation. The build-up of cholesterol eventually leads to narrowing and sometimes blockade of the blood vessels. The narrowing of the blood vessels often leads to elevated blood pressure. If a blockage happens in the arteries, main veins or the brain vessels, an outcome can be a heart attack or a stroke, and even death.

Bone & joint problems - chronic inflammation can often result in damage to the joints and bones. Osteoarthritis, rheumatoid arthritis, back problems, osteoporosis are all a result of chronic inflammation. Researchers claim that cytokines interfere with bone regeneration which leads to its deterioration.

Depression - "A new study by the Centre for Addiction and Mental Health (CAMH) found that the measure of brain inflammation in people who were experiencing clinical depression was increased by 30 percent... A growing body of evidence suggests the role of inflammation in generating the symptoms of a major depressive episode such as low mood, loss of appetite, and inability to sleep. But what was previously unclear was whether inflammation plays a role in clinical depression independent of any other physical illness." https://www.eurekalert.org/pub_releases/2015-01/cfaa-nbe012615.php

Aggressive behaviour - research has found that people with explosive anger issues have a high marker level for C-reactive proteins.

Respiratory issues - chronic inflammation is a contributory factor in the development of such conditions as asthma, chronic bronchitis, chronic obstructive pulmonary disease, emphysema and respiratory infections. Inflammation of the respiratory tract leads to accumulation of fluid and obstruction of airways which in itself can be very dangerous.

Cancer - scientists are still unsure of how inflammation leads to cancer. The two theories are that 1. immune cells attack a tumour which in turn responds by using oxygen and nutrients to grow and 2. inflammatory response can lead to a loss of proteins involved in DNA repair which leads to its mutations and cancer cells proliferation.

Reference for information in this unit:

https://www.livescience.com/52344-inflammation.html

Module 5 - Pain and Inflammation Management Methods Used in Allopathic Medicine. Their Side-effects.

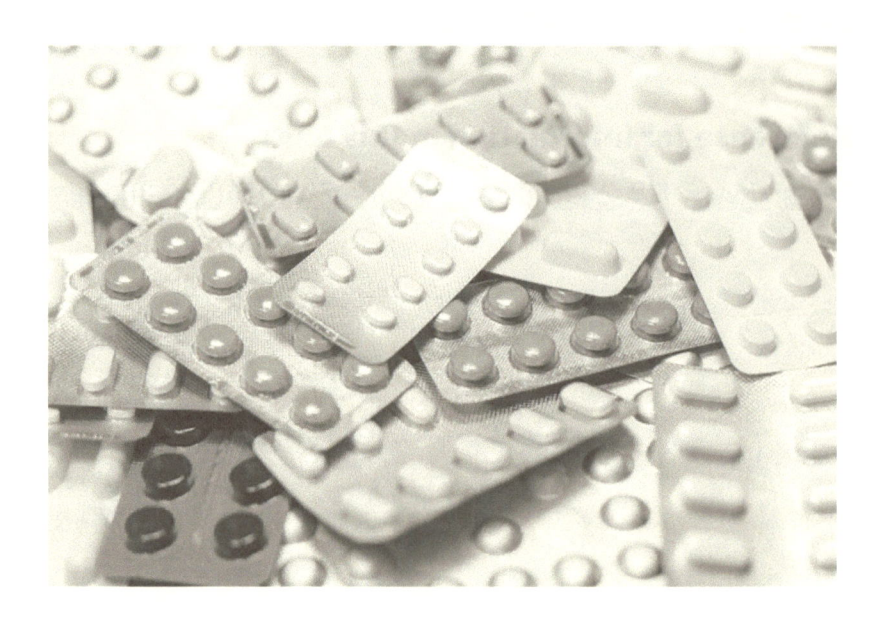

Unit 1 - Pain and Inflammation Management Methods Used in Allopathic Medicine. Side-Effects.

Allopathic (also sometimes called "traditional") medicine, or the medicine we know today, uses various remedies and procedures to address pain and inflammation. Following are the main groups of these medicines, their uses and side effects.

Paracetamol

Uses: paracetamol is an over-the-counter medicine which can be used to mild to moderate pain. It is used to address low to moderate pain and lasts up to 6 hours.

Side effects: while considered safe at recommended doses, paracetamol can be dangerous when used over a prolonged time, especially to the liver. It can also cause the following problems:

- Diarrhoea
- Profuse sweating
- Nausea
- Vomiting
- Stomach cramps
- Swelling or tenderness in the stomach area.

Overdosing on paracetamol is dangerous, so it is important not to exceed the prescribed dose.

NSAIDs

These are the drugs which reduce pain, fever and inflammation. They include aspirin, andadin, ibuprofen, naproxen, ketoprofen.

Uses: pain and inflammation relief.

Side effects: these depend on the specific drug used, but generally they include an increased risk of stomach ulceration and bleeding, heart and kidney problems, diarrhoea, IBS, liver problems, ringing in the ears, headaches, dizziness, photosensitivity and many other issues.

COX-2 inhibitors

Derived from NSAIDs, These drugs (such as rofecoxib, celecoxib, and etoricoxib) are equally effective analgesics when compared with NSAIDs, but cause less gastrointestinal haemorrhage in particular. Still, the danger is there, as seen from the side effects section.

Side effects: "May increase the risk of serious, even fatal stomach and intestinal *adverse* reactions, such as ulcers, bleeding, and perforation of the stomach or intestines."
https://www.medicinenet.com/cox-2_inhibitors/article.htm

Steroids

These are also called corticosteroids. They come in tablets, nasal sprays, inhalers, injections, lotions and creams. Some examples include prednisolone, dexamethasone and betamethasone.

"Steroids are a man-made version of hormones normally produced by the adrenal glands, two small glands found above the kidneys.

When taken in doses higher than the amount your body normally produces, steroids reduce redness and swelling (inflammation). This can help with inflammatory conditions such as asthma and eczema.

Steroids also reduce the activity of the immune system, the body's natural defence against illness and infection."
https://www.nhs.uk/conditions/steroids/

Uses: they are used to treat inflammatory conditions, such as asthma, hayfever, eczema, tennis elbow, runner's knee, frozen shoulder, ruptured disc, lupus, Crohn's disease, rheumatoid arthritis, multiple sclerosis and other similar conditions.

Side effects: used for a short time, they don't have serious side effects. However, with prolonged use they can cause indigestion, heartburn, increased appetite, weight gain, difficulty sleeping, high blood sugar/diabetes, osteoporosis, high blood pressure, weakening of the immune system, depression and suicidal thoughts.

Medical marijuana

This is a prescription drug which is a dried marijuana plant used to reduce pain and inflammation.

Opioids

Opioids are substances which act on opioid receptors in the brain to produce a morphine-like effect. In medicine, they are used for pain relief including during surgery. They include opium and morphine. There are also synthetic opioids, such as fentanyl, oxycodone and hydrocodone. Sometimes they are also referred to as narcotics.

Uses: pain relief, suppression of diarrhoea, cough, as well as replacement therapy for opioid use disorder.

Side effects: sedation, nausea, breathing difficulties, constipation, euphoria. Long-term use requires higher doses, and overdosing is not uncommon.

Opioid abuse has become a big problem in the West, especially in the US. Here are some statistics:

- "The US makes up 5 percent of the world's population and consumes approximately 80 percent of the world's prescription opioid drugs.

- Prescription opioid drugs contribute to 40 percent of all US opioid overdose deaths.
- In 2016, more than 46 people died each day from overdoses involving prescription opioids.
- Prescription opioid overdose rates are highest among people ages 25 to 54 years."
https://talbottcampus.com/prescription-drug-abuse-statistics/

There is a large percentage of people who take them for their purposes which don't involve pain management. But even when they are taken for pain, there is a high risk of getting addicted to these powerful drugs.

Conclusion

Medical painkillers, although powerful and effective, have a lot of side effects some of which can have a long-term impact on health. This calls for non-medical ways to manage pain and inflammation, and magnesium salts combined with far-infrared provide a very good alternative.

Module 6 - Far Infrared Rays - How They Work. Therapeutic Benefits & Uses.

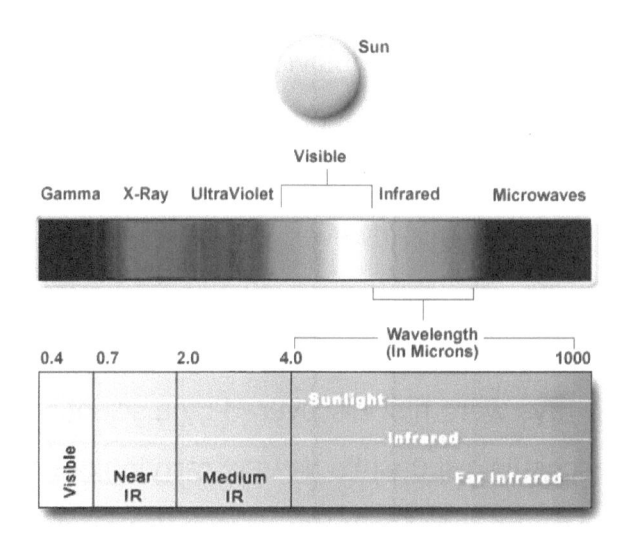

Unit 1 - Far Infrared Energy - How It Works. How FIR Interacts with the Body.

Infrared light is emitted or absorbed by molecules when they are activated by the sun. The sunlight spectrum consists of visible and invisible rays. The visible rays are what we can see when we look at a rainbow. They are red, orange, yellow, green, indigo, blue and violet. The invisible rays include ultra-violet, x-rays, gamma, cosmic, microwave, longwave, electrical wave and infrared.

The wavelength of infrared rays is between 0.76 and 1000 microns. Infrared rays are subdivided into Near (0.76-1.5 microns wavelength), Medium (1.5-4 microns) and Far Infrared (4-1000 microns). As we can see, Far Infrared has the longest wavelength. However, only a small spectrum of it is useful to life - the spectrum between 6-14 microns.

Far Infrared rays were first discovered by a scientist Sir William Herschel in 1800 while he was carrying out research; he found that Far Infrared rays were a spectrum of sunlight which existed in between visible light and microwaves. Infrared rays are invisible to the eye but can be felt by the body as heat. It is natural energy produced by the sun – about 80% of it.

Infrared has longer wavelengths than those of visible light - between 700 nanometers (nm) to 1 mm. It was discovered in 1800 by astronomer William Herschel, who discovered a type of invisible radiation in the light spectrum beyond red light, using its effect on a thermometer.

Slightly more than half of the total energy from the Sun was eventually found to arrive on Earth in the form of infrared. The recent studies have shown that Far Infrared rays emitted at 6-14 microns wavelength played an important part in the formation and development of life on Earth. The balance between absorbed and emitted infrared radiation has a critical effect on Earth's climate. On the surface of Earth, almost all thermal radiation consists of infrared rays of various wavelengths.

Infrared light has many uses - industrial, military, scientific, medical, and others. It is used in night vision devices, thermal imaging devices, astronomy, search operations, weather forecasting. The most important physical property of FI rays is their ability to be absorbed by living organisms and be harmonised with the bio-resonance life force released by the body.

How does FI energy interact with the body?

The body doesn't only absorb FI heat - it transmits it to the cells, including blood cells, to promote circulation and metabolic processes. Water molecules are affected by FI radiation, with the vibration inside the water molecule being aligned with the vibration of the FI rays.

Since 70% of the human body consists of water, it becomes a superb conductor of this energy, with water molecules in the body getting directly affected by FI rays. We have all tasted the water which we call "fresh". This is what it tastes like when it is affected by Far Infrared radiation. Infrared light is emitted or absorbed by molecules when they change their rotational-vibrational movements.

1. Far infrared gets absorbed by the skin.
2. The heat then spreads to the deeper tissues - as deep as 10 inches deep inside the body.
3. The affected body cells become energised and activated. This promotes blood flow and metabolic activities inside the body.

Among the whole spectrum of the sun rays, the Far Infrared Rays are the safest and benefit us the most. The visible light spectrum, with very short wavelengths, is reflected by the body.

Far Infrared Magnesium Wrap Course - Galina St George

The difference between far Infrared Rays (FIR) and Near Infrared rays (NIR) is that when near-infrared (NIR) waves warm up the surface it gets hot, and the heat is gradually passed on to underlying tissues through conduction. By contrast, far-infrared penetrates deeply from the beginning, so the heat gets deep into the body tissues.

The human body produces far-infrared heat naturally. The intensity of it constantly fluctuates. When it is high, our body functions to its fullest capacity. Low intensity is an indicator that the body is not 100% healthy and that the cells are not producing sufficient energy. This means that we are subject to attacks of illness and tend to age more quickly.

Far Infrared stimulates cellular metabolism which increases the ability of the body to heal itself more efficiently. It also helps to restore the functioning of the nervous system. When any tissue in the body is exposed to far-infrared rays, the healing processes are activated.

Studies suggest Far Infrared Energy helps to maintain general health and prevent disease. Far infrared rays can penetrate deep into the body, gently expanding capillaries and promoting blood circulation. This, in turn, helps to deliver nutrients and oxygen to the cells and remove toxic substances – organic and inorganic toxins. This helps to restore health and rejuvenate the body tissues inside and out.

Medical professionals in the Far East (Japan, China), Russia, Canada and other countries are using far infrared systems to rehabilitate and treat various medical problems. Far infrared heat has been known to sports therapists worldwide for its restorative ability on the muscles and joints. For example, it is used in infrared saunas to heat the occupants. Far infrared is also gaining popularity as a safe heat therapy method of natural healthcare and physiotherapy. We will talk more about it in the following unit.

Further Reading

1. The Electromagnetic Spectrum.

http://science.hq.nasa.gov/kids/imagers/ems/infrared.html

2. Far Infrared Saunas for Treatment of Cardiovascular Risk Factors.

http://www.ncbi.nlm.nih.gov/pmc/articles/PMC2718593/

3. Far infrared radiation (FIR): its biological effects and medical applications.

http://www.ncbi.nlm.nih.gov/pmc/articles/PMC3699878/

Unit 2 - Therapeutic Benefits and Uses of Far Infrared

Far Infrared energy is very important in terms of maintaining life on Earth. It plays a vital role in the hatching of an egg, and the development of a foetus of all living creatures. This means the development of organs, the circulatory system, and the formation of new cells. Without far infrared energy body cells simply could not reproduce.

To survive and thrive, a cell needs water, oxygen, nutrients and energy to be delivered to it regularly. It also needs waste materials to be removed from it regularly and efficiently. This allows cells to turn nutrients into energy and building materials for the body - blood cells, hormones, new cells to replace the old ones, etc. All this is made possible thanks to the circulatory system which acts similar to a pipeline.

When there is a blockage in it, nutrients, water and oxygen delivery and waste products removal become impeded. This leads to all sorts of health problems within the body, and in the worst cases - even death.

Since its vibrational characteristics of far infrared are in tune with the those of living cells, it is absorbed by the skin via the process of radiation, going deep into the body tissues, stimulating blood vessels and boosting circulation, which helps to deliver nutrients, oxygen and water and remove products of metabolism, CO_2 and toxic waste. The toxin removal function of FIR is very important, and this is why far infrared is used extensively in detoxification procedures.

So, what are the therapeutic benefits of Far Infrared energy?

1. **It promotes the detoxification of the body tissues.**

This is achieved through perspiration as a result of warming up of the tissues. To cool itself down, the body releases water in the form of sweat which brings to the surface products of metabolism and toxic waste. To add to this, an increase in blood circulation leads to an increase in lymph drainage, which plays the main role in detoxification, alongside perspiration.

2. **It speeds up metabolism promoting weight loss**. The warming up of body tissues means that nutrients and oxygen are delivered to the tissues at a faster rate, while products of metabolic activity and CO_2 are eliminated faster too. This means that metabolic processes in the cells happen at a faster speed, which in turn speeds up energy consumption. It leads to the body using the energy of fat cells. Since fat cells contain a lot of water and tend to store toxins, the combination of sweating and faster metabolic activity leads to release of both, and this, in turn, makes it easier for the body to use the energy of stored fat cells.

3. **It strengthens the immune system** by stimulating the production of white blood cells. This happens as a result of the tissues being warmed up which speeds up

blood circulation and white cell production. This helps to kill bacteria, viruses and fungi.

4. **FIR heat helps alleviate fatigue**, by increasing circulation and metabolism. This helps to raise vitality & feeling of well-being.

5. Helps to **eliminate lactic acid** in the body which leads to **muscle relaxation, alleviation of pain and cramps**. This is especially important after prolonged physical activity like sports exercises.

6. **It helps to reduce inflammation, chronic aches and pains. T**his happens as a result of increased circulation, removal of toxins, cellular regeneration and healing of affected tissues.

7. **FIR helps to restore healthy pH.** Again, it happens because of an increase in circulation and elimination of acid-producing toxic waste.

8. **It helps to reduce cholesterol levels** - as a result of an increase in circulation and metabolic activity.

9. **It promotes good sleep.** General relaxation involves relaxation of nerve tissues, which leads to better sleep.

10. **FIR leads to mental relaxation, relief of anxiety and depression.**

11. **It promotes tissue regeneration**, which helps to revitalise the appearance and restore skin elasticity, making it look younger and more radiant.

12. **It helps to keep the respiratory system in good health** and restore it after an illness.

There are many more conditions which Far Infrared can help with. It all comes to its ability to resonate with and work in harmony with the body.

Conditions which benefit from the use of Far Infrared:

- Heavy metal toxicity
- Other types of toxicity
- Lethargy, fatigue

- Muscle tension
- Back pain
- Cramps
- Arthritis
- Aches, pains
- Rheumatism
- High Cholesterol Level
- Diabetes
- Back problems
- Sports injuries
- Respiratory ailments - chest colds, asthma, bronchitis
- Digestive disorders
- Poor circulation
- Poor immunity, frequent infections
- Psychological stress, nervous tension
- Anxiety
- Insomnia.

Thanks to its properties, Far Infrared is used in various therapeutic devices, including saunas, blankets, mats, heaters, lamps, as well as devices for various parts of the body.

Further Reading

1. Health Benefits of Far Infrared.
http://www.clearheatersystem.co.uk/images/health_benefits_of_far_infrared_-_version_21-09-2014_.pdf
2. Far Infrared Sauna, Dr Mark Sircus.
http://drsircus.com/medicine/light-heat/far-infrared-sauna

Module 7 - Importance of Magnesium for Health. What Causes Magnesium Deficiency, and Why It Is Dangerous to Health.

Unit 1 - Importance of Magnesium for Health

Why Is Magnesium So Important to Us?

Few minerals attract as much attention as magnesium. Not only does it take part in over 300 biochemical reactions in the body but it also helps to maintain normal muscle and nerve function, steady heart rhythm, normal blood pressure, healthy immune system, strong bones and a stable blood sugar level. It also plays a big role in preventing heart disease, diabetes, cancer, osteoporosis and a whole range of other dangerous and debilitating diseases.

Magnesium is the fourth most abundant mineral in the body. About half of the total body magnesium is found in bones. The other half is found mostly inside cells of body tissues and organs. Only 1% of magnesium is found in the blood where it plays a vital role, so the body works very hard to keep the blood magnesium levels constant.

"... An important participant in enzyme processes which ensure protein biosynthesis and carbohydrate metabolism. It is also very important for the nervous and muscular systems, helps to maintain the healthy tone of the blood vessels. Magnesium is a 'calming' element for the nervous system slowing down the brain activity. It expands the blood vessels and is a natural diuretic. Generally, it is vital for all body systems and processes.

An adult requirement in magnesium is 350-500mg per day. Fresh green vegetables, seafood, soybeans, special nutritional yeasts, seeds, apples and whole grains are rich sources." Read more about the role of magnesium in the body.

Magnesium has been found to:

- Stimulate protein/fat metabolism
- Reduce inflammation by lowering the levels of histamine and serotonin (mediators of inflammation)

- Speed up rehabilitation processes in the body
- Increase testosterone levels and sperm production
- Strengthen immunity
- Slow down ageing
- Reduce cholesterol levels in the blood
- Improve the functioning of the musculoskeletal system
- Reduce blood pressure
- Significantly reduce heart disease and mortality
- Lower the incidence of cancers
- Improve the functioning of the Nervous System
- Reduce the effects of stress
- Increase phagocytosis
- Speed up tissue regeneration
- Improve skin condition
- Speed up body metabolism
- Raise energy levels (magnesium is the essential mineral in the production of energy)
- Promote weight loss

It has been proved to be a:

- Sedative

- Anti-inflammatory
- Bactericidal / fungicidal
- Circulation booster
- Analgesic
- Immune regulator.

What Happens When We Become Magnesium-Deficient?

Magnesium deficiency is more common than we realise. According to American nutritionists, an average adult needs 200mg more magnesium per day than what is obtained from the diet. The fact is that the dietary magnesium is not sufficient in providing the body with this important mineral. Magnesium deficiency can be explained by various factors, with the main reasons being depletion of soil in minerals.

"Early signs of magnesium deficiency include loss of appetite, nausea, vomiting, fatigue, and weakness. As magnesium deficiency worsens, numbness, tingling, muscle contractions and cramps, seizures, personality changes, abnormal heart rhythms, and coronary spasms can occur."
Source

Magnesium deficiency may also lead to:

- Loss of energy
- Slowing down of metabolism
- Disturbance in calcium and potassium balance in the blood
- High cholesterol level
- Formation of cholesterol plaque
- Kidney and gallbladder stones
- Arthritis
- Anxiety
- Depression
- Muscle tension
- Joint pain
- Acidosis
- Nervous tension
- Insomnia
- Diabetes
- Osteoporosis
- Chronic fatigue
- Poor immunity
- Menstrual pain

- Fertility problems.

Further Reading

1. Magnesium.
http://www.traceminerals.com/research/magnesium.htm
2. Magnesium.
http://ods.od.nih.gov/factsheets/magnesium.asp
3. Magnesium.
http://umm.edu/health/medical/altmed/supplement/magnesium

Unit 2 - What Causes Magnesium Deficiency, and Why It Is Dangerous to Health

What causes magnesium deficiency?

Magnesium deficiency is commonly caused by and associated with the following factors:

- Stress - physical and mental.

- Certain medications (e.g. insulin, diuretics, some asthma medications, birth control pills, corticosteroids, blood pressure control medicines, etc).
- Extreme physical training.
- Chemical toxins getting into the body from the environment.
- Excessive intake of sodium chloride (table salt), sugar, caffeine, alcohol, nicotine, cocaine, fizzy drinks (especially colas).
- Prolonged intense sweating, due to exercise or illness.
- Diarrhoea.
- Malnutrition. This involves not only insufficient food intake but also the consumption of nutrient-poor foods.
- Consuming food products which come from magnesium-deficient soils.
- Drinking water high in potassium.
- Prolonged physical exercise.
- Diabetes.
- Obesity.
- Kidney disease.

- Malabsorption. This can be due to compromised levels of enzymes, or unhealthy condition of the gut.
- Digestive disorders.
- Crohn's disease.
- Chemotherapy and radiotherapy.
- Liver disease.
- Inflammation.
- Serious injuries.
- Pancreatitis.
- Severe burns.

Dangers to health

So how does magnesium deficiency can affect us? Here are some conditions which may develop as a result:

- **Anxiety and panic attacks.** Magnesium helps to keep hormones in balance, and adrenal stress under control.
- **Depression.** Serotonin - the hormone responsible for mood regulation - is dependent on magnesium levels being at an optimal level in the body at all times.

- **Detoxification.** Removal of toxic elements such as lead and aluminium from the body requires the presence of sufficient levels of magnesium.
- **Diabetes.** Magnesium is needed for insulin secretion, to help metabolise sugar. Without magnesium insulin cannot transfer glucose into cells, which leads to the build-up of both glucose and insulin in the blood, leading to tissue damage.
- **Metabolic syndrome.** This condition is partly due to insufficient magnesium levels in the body, which leads to insulin not being activated, glucose not delivered to the body cells, and energy not being produced. This slows down the body metabolism.
- **Obesity.** This is also partly a result of magnesium deficiency, due to malnutrition and slow metabolism. To add to this, there is a permanent cycle of anxiety-triggered overeating, which is both caused by and leads to magnesium deficiency. Of course, one cannot just blame a low magnesium level for obesity, but it plays a big role in developing the condition.
- **Constipation.** Magnesium deficiency causes slowing down of bowel movement and constipation, which

leads to an increase of toxicity and nutrient deficiency.
- **Muscle cramps.** Magnesium is the ultimate natural relaxant. Without sufficient magnesium in the blood calcium takes over, leading to calcification of tissues and cramps.
- **Musculoskeletal problems.** Aches, pains, muscle tension are all made worse where there is not enough magnesium is present in the body. This happens due to insufficient relaxation of the muscles, which can lead to chronic tension, joint problems, inflammation and other musculoskeletal conditions, such as back problems, osteoarthritis, frozen shoulder, RSA, and more.
- **Osteoporosis.** Blood contains both calcium and magnesium, and a healthy ratio (approximately 2:1) is important to ensure bone health. Contrary to popular belief, just taking calcium and vitamin D, without supplementing magnesium, may worsen the condition, and lead to other problems.
- **Tooth decay.** Insufficient magnesium causes an imbalance of phosphorus and calcium in the saliva, which leads to tooth decay.

- **Blood clots.** Magnesium plays an important role in keeping the blood thin. Magnesium deficiency leads to thickening of the blood, and formation of blood clots, which is a potentially fatal condition.
- **Arterial plaque/ atherosclerosis.** Magnesium is necessary to keep the optimal calcium-magnesium ratio in the blood. When there is not enough magnesium, this ratio gets compromised, leading to the formation of arterial plaque, which consists of excessive blood calcium, proteins and fat. This is also a potentially fatal condition.
- **PMS/PMT - pre-menstrual syndrome/ tension** are often directly linked to magnesium deficiency.
- **Pre-eclampsia, eclampsia, premature contractions.** All of these dangerous conditions are directly caused by magnesium deficiency.
- **Fatigue.** Magnesium is the "energy" mineral. It is the spark needed to convert glucose into energy. Magnesium is also used in the production of many enzymes. When there is not enough magnesium in the body, energy does not get produced, leading to fatigue, sometimes chronic.

- **Hypertension (high blood pressure)**. Being a natural relaxant, magnesium is needed to keep blood vessels supple and open.
- **Heart disease.** Magnesium deficiency is often associated with heart disease. Doctors have been using magnesium injections for cardiac arrest and arrhythmia for a long time. The heart muscle, like any other muscles in the body, depends on magnesium for relaxation. Where there is not enough magnesium, it goes into spasm, which may lead to a heart attack and other dangerous conditions.
- **Hypoglycemia** - low blood sugar level. Blood sugar levels depend on sufficient levels of magnesium in the body which is needed for the regulation of insulin activity. Insufficient magnesium can lead not only to a buildup of glucose but to hypoglycemia as well.
- **Asthma.** Insufficient magnesium in the body increases bronchial spasm, as well as histamine production.
- **Allergy.** There is a direct link between magnesium deficiency and an allergic reaction since magnesium

manages histamine production and response within the body.

- **Kidney disease.** Magnesium deficiency can lead to abnormal lipid levels and blood sugar control, which can lead to kidney failure.
- **Headache & migraine.** Low magnesium levels lead to narrowing of blood vessels and muscle spasms, which can lead to restriction of blood flow to the brain. The other factor contributing to headaches and migraines is that serotonin does not get produced in sufficient amounts.
- **Nerve disorders.** Nerve tissue depends on magnesium for its health. Magnesium is needed to transmit nerve signals between the brain and other organs and tissues since it activates calcium. Insufficient magnesium leads to peripheral nerve problems, as well as dysfunctions of the central nervous system.

These are only some conditions caused by magnesium deficiency. All of them require increased and consistent magnesium supplementation, and oral supplementation is normally not enough.

Further Reading

1. Magnesium Deficiency Symptoms & Diagnosis, Mark Sircus.
http://drsircus.com/medicine/magnesium/magnesium-deficiency-symptoms-diagnosis
2. What Causes Magnesium Deficiency?
http://www.magnesiumoil.org.uk/what-causes-magnesium-deficiency/

Module 8 - Magnesium Supplementation Methods. Transdermal vs Oral Supplementation - Advantages and Disadvantages.

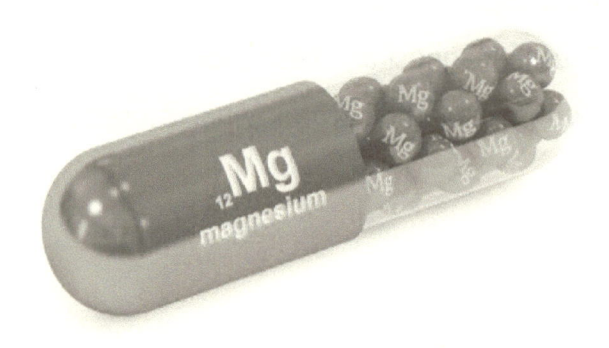

Unit 1 - Magnesium Supplementation Methods

Magnesium can be supplemented in 3 main ways: orally (tablets, milk of magnesia, capsules, powder, salt), intravenously (by injection), and transdermally (through the skin).

Some people find it difficult to tolerate oral magnesium, due to problems with their digestive system and resulting inability to absorb magnesium through intestinal walls. With magnesium being a laxative, much of it is excreted without any benefit to the body. Still, it is a method most people use - including me (alongside the transdermal one). For those who do use oral supplements, please make sure that you use chelated magnesium - not magnesium oxide since it gets into the body in an ionic form, so does not use hydrochloric acid in the stomach to break it down.

Intravenous magnesium supplementation is something which is mainly practised in a hospital environment when magnesium needs to be supplemented quickly. However, it is not a practical method for a home environment, so we won't go into detail about it.

Transdermal magnesium supplementation has proved to be very effective due to the high permeability of the skin and the fact that magnesium bypasses digestion and goes straight into the bloodstream and from there is delivered to the cells. This happens within minutes and far-infrared speeds up the process. Magnesium in salts is also easily available to the body.

Unit 2 - Transdermal vs Oral Supplementation

With so many ways to supplement magnesium, people often ask themselves a question: shall I supplement orally or transdermally? If orally (by the mouth) - which supplement is best? If transdermally - which salt shall I use?

Following is a list of various magnesium supplements, their advantages and disadvantages:

- **Magnesium oxid**e is a poorly absorbed form of magnesium since it needs to be broken down by the body, a function which falls on the stomach acid, adding a strain to the digestive system. It also can cause stool softening.

- **Magnesium chloride** and **magnesium lactate** have about 12% of magnesium but are more readily absorbed than other forms.
- **Magnesium sulphate** - take with care, as it is easy to overdose on it.
- **Magnesium** hydroxide **(milk of magnesia)** - used as a calming remedy for the stomach and a laxative. Take care to avoid overdosing.
- **Magnesium carbonate** has antacid properties, so is not suitable for everyone.
- **Magnesium glycinate (chelated form)** - has a reputation as the most efficient supplement due to the highest absorption and bioavailability. Ideal for those who aim to correct magnesium deficiency.
- **Magnesium taurate (chelated form)** - a combination of magnesium and tauric acid. Has a calming effect on the body and mind.
- **Magnesium** threonate **(chelated)** - new supplement which has a higher ability to penetrate the mitochondrial membrane, so is seen as promising.
- **Magnesium citrate (chelated)** - a combination of magnesium and citric acid. Has laxative properties.

On the other hand, **transdermal supplementation using salts such as magnesium chloride and magnesium sulphate has the following advantages:**

1. Magnesium from both salts gets absorbed by the body fast, so the effects are felt fast too.
2. There is no risk of overdosing on magnesium since the skin simply won't absorb more than the body can take.
3. The digestive system does not get involved in breaking it down. The reason oral magnesium sometimes gets poorly absorbed is that as we age, our digestive system becomes less efficient due to various factors. This impedes absorption of many nutrients, including magnesium.
4. Apart from pain relief, it offers a whole range of other benefits, which of course includes thorough relaxation, pain relief and a range of physical and psychological benefits which are being considered in the course units.

Module 9 - Products and Methods Used in Transdermal Magnesium Supplementation. Magnesium Chloride vs Magnesium Sulphate.

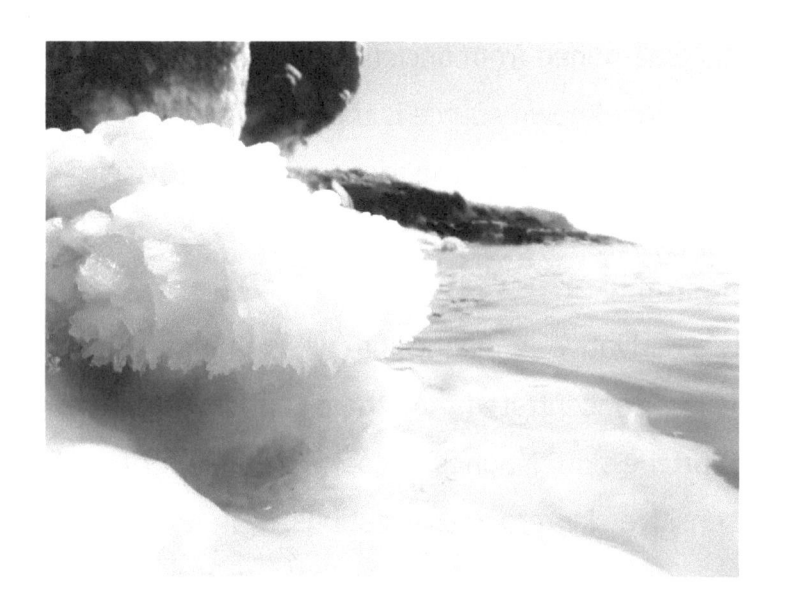

Unit 1 - Products and Methods Used in Transdermal Magnesium Supplementation

Magnesium oil

Magnesium oil is a highly concentrated salt solution which is not an oil technically but feels like a light oil to touch. Due to its oily consistency, it can be easily spread on the body. The best magnesium oil is the one which is produced from the salt mined from ancient underground deposits. The most well-known source is the Zechstein underground deposit which covers a large area in Europe, Russia.

Magnesium Gel

This is a derivative of magnesium oil, with a gel element in it. It is less concentrated than the oil and is, therefore, milder on the skin. Magnesium gel is suitable for people with sensitive skin prone to irritations.

Magnesium Flake

Magnesium flake is crystallized magnesium chloride. It still contains water - this is why it is called Magnesium Chloride Hexahydrate - but in a much slammer concentration than magnesium oil.

You can make magnesium oil from a flake. Mix 1 part of magnesium flake with 1 part of hot water. If the flake won't mix, warm up the mixture, and add more water. Alternatively, use it in a bath/ foot bath.

Epsom Salt

It is another name for Magnesium Sulphate. Epsom salt can be used in a bath, foot bath, or body wrap.

Methods of Transdermal Magnesium Supplementation

- Applying magnesium oil on the body by hand
- Spraying magnesium oil on the body
- Bath - with magnesium chloride or magnesium sulphate
- Footbath
- Compress
- Body wrap.

Further Reading

1. How to Replenish Magnesium Level in the Body & Keep It High. http://www.magnesiumoil.org.uk/how-to-replenish-magnesium-level-in-the-body-quickly-keep-it-high/

2. Magnesium Oil Massage. http://www.magnesiumoil.org.uk/magnesium-oil-massage/

3. Magnesium Oil Compress. http://www.magnesiumoil.org.uk/magnesium-chloride-compress/

Unit 2 - Magnesium Chloride vs Magnesium Sulphate

I have been asked many times about the **differences between magnesium chloride and magnesium sulphate**, *commonly known as* **Epsom Salts**. *There is a great article about it written by Dr Mark Sircus, a well-know and recognised researcher of magnesium and its benefits. I quote it here:*

"According to Daniel Reid, author of The Tao of Detox, magnesium sulfate, commonly known as Epsom salts, is rapidly excreted through the kidneys and therefore difficult to assimilate. This would explain in part why the effects from Epsom salt baths do not last long and why you need more magnesium sulfate in a bath than magnesium chloride to get similar results. Magnesium chloride is easily assimilated and metabolized in the human body.[1] However, Epsom salts are used specifically by parents of children with autism because of the sulfate, which they are usually deficient in, sulfate is also crucial to the body and is wasted in the urine of autistic children.

For purposes of cellular detoxification and tissue purification, the most effective form of magnesium is magnesium chloride, which has a strong excretory effect on toxins and stagnant energies stuck in the tissues of the body, drawing them out through the pores of the skin. This is powerful hydrotherapy that draws toxins from the tissues, replenishes the "vital fluid" of the cells and restores cellular magnesium to optimum levels. Magnesium Chloride is environmentally safe and is used around vegetation and in agriculture. It is not irritating to the skin at lower concentrations and is less toxic than common table salt.

Magnesium Chloride solution was not only harmless for tissues, but it had also a great effect over leucocytic activity and phagocytosis; so it was perfect for external wounds treatment.

Dr Jean Durlach et al, at the Université P. et M. Curie, Paris, wrote a paper about the relative toxicities between magnesium sulfate and magnesium chloride. They write, "The reason for the toxicity of magnesium pharmacological doses of magnesium using the sulfate anion rather than the chloride anion may perhaps arise from the respective chemical structures of both the two magnesium salts. Chemically, both $MgSO_4$ and $MgCl_2$ are hexa-aqueous complexes. However $MgCl_2$ crystals consist of dianions with magnesium coordinated to the six water molecules as a complex, $[Mg(H_2O)_6]^{2+}$ and two independent chloride anions, Cl^-. In $MgSO_4$, a seventh water molecule is associated with the sulphate anion, $[Mg(H_2O)_6]^{2+}[SO_4.H_2O]$. Consequently, the more hydrated $MgSO_4$ molecule may have chemical interactions with paracellular components, rather than with cellular components, presumably potentiating toxic manifestations while reducing therapeutic effect."

MgSO4 is not always the appropriate salt in clinical therapeutics. MgCl2 seems the better anion-cation association to be used in many clinical and pharmacological indications.[2] Dr Jean Durlach et al.

Magnesium sulfate is a chemical compound containing magnesium and sulfate, with the formula $MgSO_4$. In its hydrated form, the pH is 6.0 (5.5 to 7.0). It is often encountered as the heptahydrate, $MgSO_4 \cdot 7H_2O$, commonly called Epsom salts. Anhydrous magnesium sulfate is used as a drying agent. Since the anhydrous form is hygroscopic (readily absorbs water from the air) and therefore harder to weigh accurately, the hydrate is often preferred when preparing solutions, for example in medical preparations. Epsom salts have traditionally been used as a component of bath salts.

References:

[1] http://www.hps-online.com/foodprof14.htm
[2] Magnesium Research. Volume 18, Number 3, 187-92, September 2005, original article"

http://magnesiumforlife.com/product-information/magnesium-chloride-vs-magnesium-sulfate/

Far Infrared Magnesium Wrap Course - Galina St George

Module 10 - Managing Pain Using Far Infrared and Magnesium

Unit 1 - Managing Pain Using Far Infrared

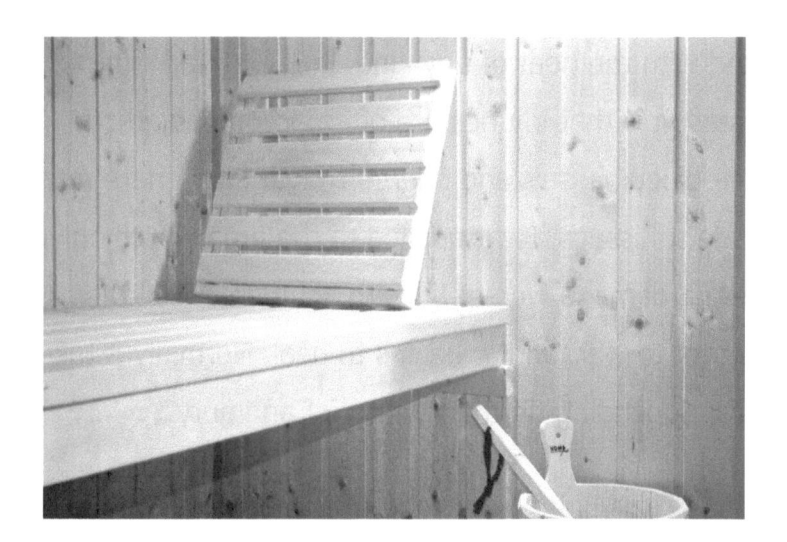

Unlike near-infrared, far infrared rays penetrate deep into the body tissues. This means that it can address the areas of pain hidden deep inside the body.

Of course, if it is undiagnosed pain of unknown origin, one should always seek medical diagnosis and advice. However, when pain is linked to muscle, tendon, joint or nerve tissue damage, cramps or stomach spasms which have been medically diagnosed, far infrared can be of great benefit if used properly and in good time.

One needs to remember that a fresh injury should never be treated with the heat of any kind, including far-infrared. The reason is that injuries are often accompanied by broken blood vessels and haemorrhage. Plus, there may be damage to tissues. Heat applied to the area would only make the damage worse. So with acute injuries, it is important to wait until it begins to heal. Normally it takes 2-3 days, depending on the severity of an injury.

You can start using the heat once the acute pain and inflammation have gone (it depends on how severe the damage is). Once you feel that the injury is beginning to heal, far-infrared heat can be used in the area. It's preferable to ordinary convection heat since it would go deep inside the body and stimulate tissue recovery. Never apply any kind of heat on an inflamed area which is warmer than the surrounding tissues and is acutely painful. It normally means that healing hasn't started yet.

Far infrared works well on spasms and cramps. The heat goes deep into the tissues relaxing them. This stimulates the blood flow to the area resulting in further relaxation, spasm and cramp relief.

It's best not to use far infrared if you have a period pain since it can make the bleeding worse. In such cases I would suggest just applying magnesium oil on the area and perhaps using a hot water bottle which is just a little bit above the body temperature, to bring relief from the spasm.

Far infrared used on areas of nerve pain, such as sciatica or "twisted" back, can also bring great relief. It should also be used with great care, on lower settings, since sciatica involves inflammation.

So how does far infrared help with pain?

- It warms up hardened tissues and tight muscles relaxing them as a result.
- It flushes the substances which cause inflammation from the area.
- It speeds up recovery by increasing metabolism in the area.
- It works on a deep tissue level rather than superficially thus increasing the possibility and speed of recovery.
- By warming the tissues, it works on a psychological level as well as physical.

As you can see, far infrared works well by dealing with pain on its own. Adding magnesium salts would make it many times more effective.

Unit 2 - Managing Pain Using Magnesium

Magnesium is one of the most powerful natural relaxants in nature. It also has a profound effect on the functioning of the nervous system. Without sufficient magnesium, nerves start firing signals too easily with even a minor stimulus. Noises become too loud, lights too bright, emotions exaggerated. Magnesium is known to regulate or inhibit many nerve receptors. It acts like water on a fire, cooling down the nervous system.

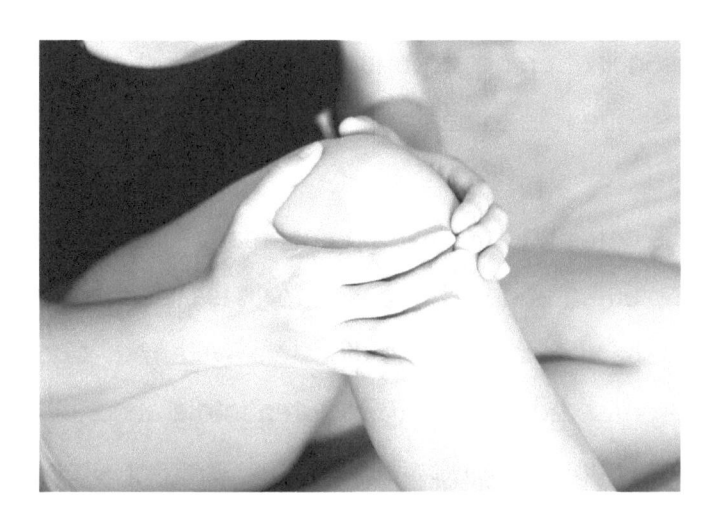

Magnesium also affects the nervous system by regulating the release of hormones, which occurs due to many different forms of stress. "Without enough magnesium, serotonin flows unchecked, constricting blood vessels and releasing other pain-producing chemicals such as substance P and prostaglandins, he says. Normal magnesium levels not only prevent the release of these pain-producing substances but also stop their effects, says Dr Altura."
http://www.mgwater.com/prev1801.shtml

Unfortunately, it is very difficult to determine magnesium deficiency using a blood test, since blood serum level does not reflect the amount of magnesium in the tissues. This is the reason it often gets overlooked, and unnoticed, with dire consequences to health.

Also, it is difficult to achieve optimal magnesium levels via oral supplementation. The reason for it is that magnesium is not easily absorbed by the digestive system. If digestion is compromised due to an IBS, gluten intolerance, or leaky gut, then supplementation becomes an even greater challenge. To add to it a diet high in processed foods which contain phosphates, and much of oral magnesium will pass through the body unabsorbed.

Further Reading

1. Inflammation & Pain Management with Magnesium. http://drsircus.com/medicine/magnesium/inflammation-and-systemic-stress

2. Magnesium Treats Fibromyalgia Pain.
http://www.fmnetnews.com/latest-news/magnesium-treats-fibromyalgia-pain

Module 11 - Far Infrared Magnesium Pain and Health Management Wrap

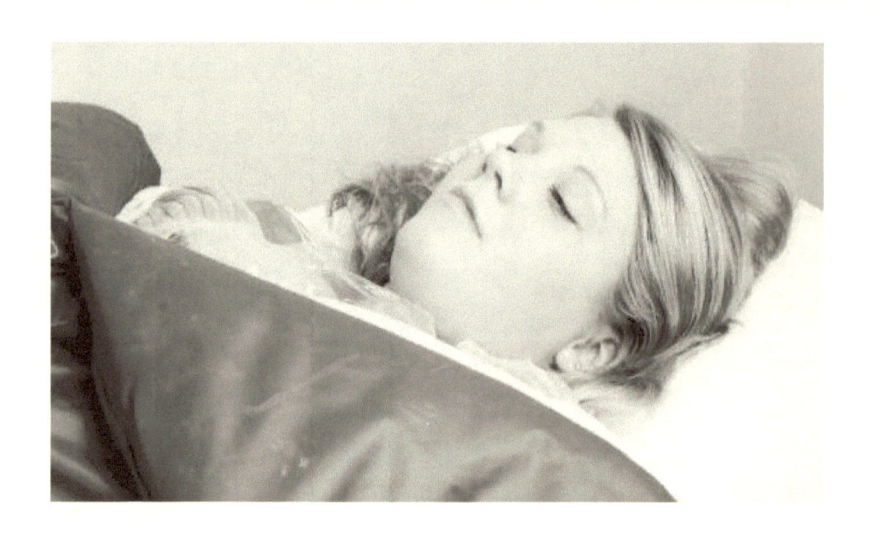

Unit 1 - FIR Magnesium Pain and Health Management Wrap - Benefits, Uses, Contraindications, Cautions

Benefits

There are numerous benefits which Far Infrared Magnesium Wraps can offer. We have already listed the health benefits of far-infrared heat and transdermal magnesium applications. Used together, far-infrared heat and magnesium have the potential to produce really powerful results. Following are just some of the benefits of the treatment.

Detoxification

Achieved through activation of the body cells, profound sweating due to far-infrared heat which stimulates the removal of toxins, boosted by the powerful detoxifying properties of the minerals.

Water retention

Lymphatic drainage is activated as a result of stimulation of the blood flow, which helps drain water from where it has been stagnant - mostly the extremities, such as legs and arms.

Sluggish metabolism

The wraps promote cellular activity as a result of the speed-up of circulation. Increased blood flow to the cells helps to deliver nutrients and remove products of metabolic activity much faster.

Weight loss

The treatment leads to profuse sweating and speeding up of metabolic activity, as well as higher energy levels. This helps to kick-start weight loss. It should, of course, be used in conjunction with exercise and a healthy diet.

Skin rejuvenation

The treatment promotes cellular activity and regeneration, which results in skin rejuvenation - it can be noticed even after the first treatment.

Stress reduction

The treatment relaxes all the body tissues and systems, including nervous. Magnesium is a powerful natural relaxant, and so is the infrared heat. This leads to profound relaxation of the body and mind.

Relief from aches & pains

Achieved through relaxation of the muscles and nervous tissues.

Uses

General Detox
Far Infrared stimulates the activity of all the body tissues, on a very deep level. Where the body is heated normally, it would eliminate toxins mainly from the superficial layers of the skin. With infrared heat, deep layers of the skin and body tissues are stimulated into releasing toxins. The blood vessels expand, and this promotes blood circulation, which speeds up nutrient/toxin exchange. Detoxification using Far Infrared systems becomes much more effective and speedier.
Using magnesium chloride or Epsom salt helps to supplement magnesium levels in the body, which in turn helps to produce the energy required for detoxification.

Alcohol & Drugs Detox

Far Infrared has an incredible ability to stimulate all the body tissues and promote detoxification. This can make it a great aid for those undergoing a drugs/ alcohol detox programme. Magnesium is a highly deficient element in people using alcohol and drugs. Far Infrared Magnesium Wrap will help to both stimulate the cells into releasing toxins and provide the body with magnesium it so desperately needs. A series of treatments would be needed in this case, and they should always be observed by a medical practitioner. Don't attempt to do it if you are not a medical professional.

Weight Loss

Because of their ability to speed up cellular metabolism, detoxification and remove excess water in the body, FIR systems are increasingly used in weight management. The effects are so powerful that they can be experienced instantly. A person feels much lighter even after one treatment, although it would be mainly water that they would have lost in a single treatment.

The systems have to be used in conjunction with sensible eating and exercise, although having treatments would greatly boost the body's ability to detoxify itself and remove that excess water and toxins from the fatty tissues which often make weight loss a difficult issue. Far Infrared is a great aid which makes the process of weight loss easier, more pleasant and fun.

Pain Management - Sport and Other Applications

Far Infrared gently relaxes all the body tissues, and this helps relieve muscle tension, improve blood circulation in stagnant areas of the body relieving accumulation of lactic acid which is a major source of pain in sportspeople and those suffering from gout for example, and also a large majority of people who live stressful lives and do not have time to look after their nutrition and health.

Using FIR heat helps promote a healthy pH in the body. For sportspeople Far Infrared is a great way to restore muscles and joints, and recover from injuries at a much faster pace then they would otherwise. Adding magnesium to the treatment helps to relax the tissues even further, due to the powerful relaxing properties of magnesium and the ability of the skin to absorb it.

Poor Immunity

FIR heat is naturally produced by all living organisms, and a healthy body produces a balanced amount of far-infrared heat. When we become ill, the balance is disturbed. The body naturally starts to produce more heat to fight bacteria and viruses. This is the time when it is best to leave the body to cope with infection using its resources.

However, we can boost our immune system at other times when we feel that it needs a boost – e.g. when we catch infections frequently, are feeling tired, when our energy levels go down. This creates a good environment for disease. Far Infrared heat helps boost the lymphocyte and phagocyte levels in the body and prevent an infection from taking over.

Addition of magnesium to the treatment helps to boost the immune system even further, by delivering this important element where it is most needed – to the cells - where it is used to produce energy and hormones which are responsible for the health of the immune system.

Passive Exercise

Because of the ability of Far Infrared heat to relax the tissues, gently expand the blood vessels and boost circulation, it is used in cases where exercise becomes difficult or impossible. The heat will also help to remove accumulating toxins, excess water, and boost tissue regeneration. It also has a profound psychological effect, since it promotes relaxation of the nervous tissues as well. Magnesium delivered to the cells restores energy and health, helping the person to get back to active life.

Stress Relief

Far Infrared heat penetrates deep into the body tissues, bringing a feeling of deep relaxation and comfort. Since it relaxes all the organs and body tissues, including nervous, which involves the brain, FIR has a profound psychological effect on the body. It promotes a feeling of calm and tranquillity, relieving anxiety, depression, insomnia and other effects of stress, even after one treatment. It is a must for those whose life is hectic and stressful. Magnesium, being one of the most powerful natural relaxants, promotes stress relief and relaxation even further.

Clinic & Home Use

Far Infrared systems are safe to use both in the clinic and at home in the majority of cases. There are contra-indications and cautions which should always be taken into account. However, for a large majority of people they will be a great aid to use for aches, pains, lowered immunity, insomnia, fatigue, low energy levels, water retention, weight problems.

Far infrared heat is wonderful on cold winter nights, after work when feeling cold and tired. In therapy clinics, FIR is used both in health and beauty treatments – to promote healing, reduce aches and pains, help speed up tissue regeneration and promote detoxification, excess water retention and weight loss. For a therapist, it is a great addition to the treatments they can already offer to their clients.

Other Uses

- Muscle tension
- Muscle cramps
- Poor circulation
- Osteoporosis
- Predisposition to high blood pressure
- Joint problems
- General aches and pains
- Stress-related conditions
- Fatigue
- Poor immunity
- Insomnia
- Headaches, migraines
- Irritability, anxiety
- Back, shoulder, neck aches/pains
- Sports injuries

Far Infrared Magnesium Wrap Course - Galina St George

- After-sport therapy
- Muscle cramps
- Nervous tension
- Aches, pains

Beauty

- Cellulite reduction (beauty)
- Skin rejuvenation
- As part of a weight loss programme
- Puffiness, water retention
- Body rejuvenation

Contra-Indications

- Heart disease
- Cardiovascular conditions
- Blood pressure abnormalities (high, low, unstable)
- Cancer
- Undiagnosed health conditions
- Pregnancy
- Epilepsy

- Deep vein thrombosis
- Undiagnosed lumps
- Inflammations
- Infections
- Fever
- Rheumatoid arthritis
- Asthma
- Menstruation
- Diabetes
- Being under the age of 16 (parent's permission required)
- Being under the effect of drugs and alcohol
- Ulcers
- Recent operations
- Wounds, broken skin, other non-contagious skin conditions
- Undiagnosed aches and pain
- Lymphoedema
- Bruising, recent traumas
- Fever / high temperature
- General weakness and debility
- Contagious skin disorders
- Shingles/ herpes

- Psychiatric problems
- Addictions.

This list is non-exhaustive, and there can be other contra-indications not listed here. The main thing to bear in mind is that if you are in doubt, do not do the treatment until you have received written permission from the doctor. Some of these contra-indications may still qualify the client for a treatment, but their doctor's permission is required nonetheless.

Cautions

- Chronic conditions
- Sensitive skin
- History of heart problems
- Feeling weak
- Dizziness
- Low blood pressure
- Thyroid problems
- Being on medication
- Anything which you may have doubts about.

If the client has any health problems, ask them to consult their GP and ask for written permission to have the treatment. If in doubt, do not do it. Make sure that the Consent Form has been signed by the client before commencing the treatment. You can **find more information about contraindications here.**

What to Do If the Treatment is Unsuitable for a Client

It is best to email your client a form before they come for a treatment, to avoid wasting everyone's time. However, even if you do this, you may still discover that the treatment is not suitable for a client. If you find out that this is the case, explain to your client that it is in their best interests to see their medical doctor and ask for their approval for the treatment. You will also need to let your client know that your judgment is based on their word and that it is in their best interests to tell you everything as it is. Make sure that they sign the consultation form before the treatment.

Unit 2 - Products, Materials and Equipment

If you are doing it in a therapy room or spa

You may have some of these products and materials already. These are my recommendations if you don't yet. Please note that I am an **Amazon Associate** and these are affiliate links.

1. Magnesium oil
2. Massage table
3. Massage table cover
4. Disposable plastic sheet for the wrap (I use a dust sheet for my wraps - it's easy to cut to the right body size).
5. Cotton sheet (alternative to a plastic sheet)
6. Far infrared sauna bag
7. Large towel
8. Large bowl (for warm water)
9. Couch roll
10. Headband or turban

11. Disposable panties
12. Paper towel roll
13. A soft sponge (to clean the body with)
14. Drinking water.

Preparation

- Couch – with the cover on, the infrared blanket laid out and switched on to keep it warm, and the plastic sheet laid out on top of the blanket, with the paper couch cover on top of the plastic sheet (this is to keep the client comfortable during the initial massage).
- If the shower facilities are not available, as is often the case with a majority of therapy settings, then prepare a large bowl of very warm water just before the end of the treatment, a sponge and a small towel, to clean up the client after the treatment.
- Set the control device for the FIR blanket on a moderate heat setting of about 45-50 degrees C, and the timer to 45 minutes. Set it 15 minutes before the treatment starts (so total setting will be 60 minutes), so that the blanket is warm when the client lies

down on the couch. You will need to check by feeling and checking with the client whether the blanket is being heated evenly in all parts, and doesn't overheat.
- Cover the blanket with a thin plastic sheet the size of the client's height. This protects the blanket and promotes more sweating.
- Make sure that hygiene is observed at all times. Always wash your hands before the treatment begins. Make sure that the materials and equipment are clean to avoid cross-infection.

If you are doing it at home

- Magnesium oil
- Soft mat to put on the floor (if you don't have a massage table)
- Far infrared sauna bag
- Disposable plastic sheet for the wrap
- Cotton sheet (alternative to a plastic sheet)
- Drinking water.

Preparing Magnesium Chloride Solution

Add 1 part of magnesium chloride flakes to 4 parts of very warm water. So if you have 1 litre of water, you will need to add 200g of magnesium flakes. With magnesium oil, use 1 part of magnesium oil to 2 parts of water. For example, 1 litre of water would require 330ml of magnesium. The amount of magnesium oil or flakes can be reduced if the client has sensitive skin. I suggest preparing the solution immediately before doing the wrap (after the massage), to make sure that it stays warm.

Unit 3 - Far Infrared Magnesium Wrap Procedure

Consultation

- Make sure that the client is suitable for the treatment and has no contra-indications, by taking a thorough consultation. The consultation sheet needs to include the client's health history, any past or present conditions, chronic or acute, a treatment plan, client's expectations for the treatment (make sure

they are realistic), and client's signature of consent to the treatment.
- Check that the client has no fever, that they don't suffer from high or low blood pressure or heart problems, and are not taking medication or is under the influence of drugs/ alcohol. Watch their behaviour. Check their skin condition to make sure that there are no irritations, fresh scars, scratches, inflammations, or open wounds. For a female client – ask again if she is pregnant or having a period. These would be contraindications to the treatment.
- Explain what is going to happen and how the client can expect to feel during and after treatment. Tell them that you are going to ask how they are feeling throughout the treatment. Explain the importance of hydration.
- What is their goal for the treatment (e.g. relief from back pain, joint and muscle aches and tension, weight loss, stress relief, relaxation, skin rejuvenation, etc)?
- Answer questions. Let them know that you are going to stay with them throughout the whole treatment.

Ask them to let you know if they start feeling uncomfortable at any time during the treatment. Ask them to sign the consultation form which would stipulate that they have given you all the information regarding their state of health and agree to undergo the treatment.

Treatment

- Provide disposable panties to wear, to preserve the client's modesty. Ask the client to undress and lie down on the couch which has a warmed up far-infrared blanket with a disposable plastic sheet on top. Lay the paper couch cover on top just for the massage.
- Make sure that everything is at hand to ensure a smooth flow of the treatment. It helps to have a bowl of warm water and a towel, in case you need to wash your hands during the treatment.
- Start massaging the client with a warmed-up product. The massage product can be magnesium oil or in cases of your client having sensitive skin, coconut oil or any other massage oil can be used to

create a barrier between the product and the skin. It won't reduce the absorption of magnesium ions too much but will soften the effect of the saline solution.

- Having massaged the back and the front of the body with the magnesium oil, remove the couch roll.
- Wrap the client up with the cotton sheet soaked with the magnesium oil solution.
- Wrap the plastic sheet over the client's body, and cover the client with the top part of the blanket.
- Leave the blanket loose if a client doesn't like to be restricted with fastening (some clients can be claustrophobic, so check for this).
- There will be 3 layers - cotton sheet, plastic sheet and the blanket.
- Make sure that the **temperature is comfortable** for the client. A mid-range temperature of about 50 degrees C provides gentle heat and is pleasant and effective at the same time, since it can be tolerated for a relatively long time without creating discomfort, thus prolonging the interaction of the product with the body.
- **Keep communicating** with the client throughout the treatment to make sure that they are

comfortable and not too hot or thirsty. Offer them water regularly. Never leave the room while the client is still in the bag. Make sure that they can open the bag easily and come out of it if they want to.
- The client will normally stay in the blanket for 40-45 minutes - up to an hour.
- While in the blanket, many clients want to just go to sleep. If you are qualified in reflexology or are a beauty therapist, you can offer the client a reflexology treatment or a mini-facial while they are wrapped up in the blanket. However, they may just want to lie in the blanket and enjoy the procedure as it is.

Ending the treatment

- After the treatment is finished, unwrap the client and dry them with a towel. Offer a shower if it is available.
- If a shower is not available, use a bowl of water and a sponge plus a small towel to remove the salt and clean and dry the client up.

- Spread coconut oil or cocoa butter oil on the client's skin after the shower (wash).
- Ask how they are feeling. Make sure they are not drowsy or are otherwise feeling unwell.
- Offer them to rest in the reception for 15-20 minutes to cool down and regain balance before they leave the clinic. Offer the client water or herbal tea to rehydrate, and advise them to keep drinking mineral water after the treatment.
- Clean up the equipment and the blanket. Use a disinfectant spray for the blanket, or wash it with soap and a sponge to keep it clean for the next client.

After-care, Feedback, Re-book

After-care advice: Advise the client to drink lots of water to re-hydrate (slightly salted/ mineral water), no heavy meals on the day, sleep and relaxation are essential. Explain how they may feel after the treatment - light-headed, have a slight headache, feeling tired for a while, depending on their general health condition. Explain that these are normal feelings and that they will pass eventually.

Tell them to see the doctor if they start feeling poorly, or are otherwise concerned about their condition.

Feedback: How does the client feel? Did she/he enjoy the treatment? Is there anything that he/she didn't like?

Re-book: Explain, that while a one-off treatment is beneficial, the best results can be achieved if they undertake a course of at least 4 treatments, preferably once a week. Offer discounts on block bookings. For more information, see the Marketing module.

Variation of the Treatment

Optional products

Magnesium oil is not the only product that can be used in magnesium wraps. If a person loves a scrub, then you can add some fine sea salt, Himalayan or the Dead Sea salt into magnesium oil and give the body a good scrub before the client being wrapped up. For those with sensitive skin, a gel may be used instead of the oil.

Performing the Treatment on Yourself

Is it possible to do the treatment to yourself? The short answer is: yes. How can it be done? The same way as above, except that you will need to do everything yourself, so the process will need to be simplified. For example, massaging yourself may need to be omitted, since it would be rather difficult unless you have someone around to do it for you. However, if you are on your own, proceed straight to doing the wrap.

Materials & equipment

- Far infrared blanket
- Cotton sheet
- Plastic sheet roll (wide enough to wrap yourself in) - optional
- Magnesium oil
- A spray bottle
- Large bowl
- Towel
- Cotton sheet (optional)
- Water to drink.

Procedure

- Switch on the blanket to warm it up. It normally takes about 10 minutes to warm up.
- Spread the plastic sheet on top of the blanket.
- Soak the cotton sheet in the magnesium chloride solution prepared earlier. Lay it on top of the plastic sheet.
- Lie down on top, cover yourself with the cotton sheet and the plastic sheet.
- Cover yourself with the top part of the blanket.
- Stay in the blanket for about 40-45 minutes - up to 1 hour.
- Get out of the blanket.
- Shower
- Spread coconut oil or cocoa butter all over the body
- Drink water
- Rest.

It is good to have someone present while you are having the treatment - to help with fiddly tasks (such as covering your body with magnesium and wrapping yourself in the sheets and the blanket), as well as to keep an eye on you in case you want a drink of water. But if you are in good health, it is not necessary - just an advantage.

It is also good to do this treatment before bedtime so that you can sleep afterwards. Make sure you drink plenty of water afterwards. I suggest adding a small pinch of Himalayan or sea salt to the water, to restore the salt-water balance within the body.

Performing the Treatment on Friends & Family

The treatment for yourself and family would not be different from what you do for your clients, except that there is no need for the couch since the treatment can be done on the floor (put some soft mat underneath for comfort). All the rest is the same, including, of course, checking for contra-indications.

Module 12 - Other Conditions Far Infrared Magnesium Wrap Can Help With

Unit 1 - Other Conditions Far Infrared Magnesium Wrap Can Help With

While this course focuses mainly on pain management, there are many other uses for Far Infrared Mineral Wraps. The reason for it is that both far-infrared and magnesium salts have a whole range of health benefits which can address a large number of issues. Here are just some of them:

- **Metabolic, energy & weight issues.** Magnesium plays a very important part in metabolic processes. It is needed for effective sugar, fat and protein metabolism. When we are deficient in magnesium, these processes slow down which affects our energy levels and a general state of health. We become lethargic and start gaining weight. Transdermal magnesium supplementation tops up magnesium levels fast without involving digestion. Far infrared ensures an even faster delivery to tissues deep inside the body by warming up the tissues. This makes the combination so effective for metabolism, energy and weight management.

- **Poor circulation.** Magnesium promotes relaxation of tissues and blood circulation. Far infrared has a similar effect. Together they work very efficiently to improve blood flow in the body. This is linked to improved metabolism, increased energy and weight loss promotion.
- **Cramps, muscle tension.** Relaxation of the tissues by using far-infrared and magnesium helps to relieve both cramps and muscle tension.
- **Stress, anxiety, insomnia.** Magnesium and far-infrared used together relax the Central Nervous System reducing stress, anxiety and insomnia in the process.
- **Blood sugar management.** Magnesium is a very important mineral in the prevention and treatment of diabetes. Magnesium deficiency raises the chances of developing diabetes.

- **Prevention of hypertension.** Magnesium relaxes blood vessels reducing blood pressure on them. This makes it an important factor in ensuring optimal blood pressure. However, people who are on blood pressure medication should seek medical advice before using the wrap or magnesium. The treatment can be used by those who seek to prevent developing blood pressure problems.
- **Poor immunity.** Magnesium is essential for a strong immune system. Topping up magnesium levels by using the Far Infrared Magnesium Wrap would help to strengthen immunity.
- **Ageing skin.** Using magnesium and far-infrared benefits skin enormously. It delivers magnesium to the deeper skin layers relaxing and removing excess calcium from the tissues. It also helps to improve the blood flow to the skin delivering nutrients and water and removing metabolic waste and dead skin cells. The skin looks visibly better after the procedure.
- **Improved detox.** Using far infrared helps to promote the removal of toxins from the body. Magnesium is a vital element in the detoxification

processes. Both work well together to ensure effective detox.

There are many other issues which would benefit from the use of Far Infrared Magnesium Wraps. They truly work holistically, addressing and balancing all the body systems.

Module 13 - Case studies and Practical Training

Unit 1 – Case Studies

Students who are training to offer therapies to the members of the public will be required to submit case studies on 3 clients (2 treatment for each client minimum) before a certificate of completion will be issued.

The case studies can be performed on family members, friends or other volunteers. The case studies must include a consultation form with a client's real name, address, signature and feedback. The case studies can be submitted by post, in person, or online.

The description of the treatment must include:

- Background information about the client - name, age, gender, occupation, lifestyle.
- Her/his physical condition.
- Their psychological state.

- Their goal for the treatment.
- Any existing contra-indications.
- What treatment plan has been agreed with them (how many treatments, how often, how long, what will be the focus on for the treatments).
- How each treatment went.
- How the client felt before, during and after the treatment.
- Client's feedback.
- Aftercare advice is given.

Each treatment should be recorded separately. You will need to conduct at least 2 treatments per client, 3 clients in total for certification. At the end of the course of treatments, you will need to record a general conclusion as to whether the goals for the course of treatments have been achieved. There should also be a general signed consultation form (one is enough) for the course of treatments.

See a sample description of a case study I did on a client some time ago. It relates to Sports Massage, but you will be able to see how I recorded it. I didn't include the consultation form since it contained private information, but all the data you need is in the form - all you need is to fill it in, and get the client sign it.

Unit 2 - Consultation Form

What The Consultation Form Should Include: Check List

- Client's name
- Client's address
- Client's phone number
- Doctor's name and address
- Present health condition
- Past health history
- Your observation of their physical condition and behaviour
- Contra-indications
- Cautions
- What they want to achieve with the treatment(s)
- Agreed treatment plan
- Consent form (disclaimer)

Far Infrared Magnesium Wrap Course - Galina St George

- Date
- Signature.

Make sure that you have all of these things covered, and a get them to sign the statement that they are fit for a treatment - before you commence the treatment.

Download the form below and use as it is, or change to create your own.

Download the Consultation Form - PDF format
Download the Consultation Form - Word format

Unit 3 - Practical Training

Practical training is a 2-4-hour module which is offered to therapists and members of the public. It is an option for members. UK/ Ireland therapists who would like to practise professionally and apply for 3rd party insurance are strongly advised to take it.

Our students in other countries need to make enquiries and arrangements locally regarding professional insurance, and of course, for you, the Practical module is an option.

Although for non-therapists the practical module is an option, we strongly recommend that you take it, for a better understanding of the procedures, and to get answers to any questions you may have while learning it.

Training is normally provided to 2 students at a time. However, one-to-one training is also available. You can either bring your model for the treatment or work on each other. Materials and equipment will be provided for practical training, so you don't have to bring anything for it - just a notebook and a pen.

Please email us with any questions:
support@purenaturecures.com

Further Information

Did you find information in this book useful? Leave feedback to me know what you think!
Would you like to learn more? I have published a number of books on the subject of minerals. You can find them on Amazon.

Mineral Healing Books

1. **Earth's Humble Healers:** Learn How to Use Salts, Muds & Clays for Better Health, Youth & Vitality. Plus 80 Health & Beauty Recipes
2. **How Clays Work:** Science & Applications of Clays & Clay-like Minerals in Health & Beauty
3. **Magnesium at Home:** 25 Most Common Health Conditions & How Magnesium Salts Can Help
4. **Mineral Healing Recipe Book:** An overview of how minerals can be used in everyday life to address common health problems, boost health and vitality.
5. **Introduction to Mineral Healing**
Learn interesting facts about healing properties of salts, muds, clays, zeolite and diatomaceous earth. It is a good

book to start learning about minerals.

6. **First Aid Guide to Minerals**

Find out how salts, muds and clays can help when medicines are unavailable.

Courses

1. **Far Infrared Mineral Weight Loss Wrap Course** for Clinic & Home Use: Learn how to use clays, salts and far infrared for sustainable weight loss and better health

https://www.amazon.com/dp/B07N99H1XV

2. **Far Infrared Magnesium Wrap Course for Clinic & Home Use**: Learn how to use magnesium salts and far infrared for better health and vitality

https://www.amazon.com/dp/B07JZDWQX1

3. **Transdermal Magnesium Therapy Course for Clinic & Home Use**

https://www.amazon.com/dp/B07GXXGWT7

4. **Far Infrared Clay Detox Wrap Course for Clinic & Home Use:** Learn how to use clays and far infrared for transdermal detox and healing

https://www.amazon.com/dp/B07JCL55TZ

5. **Forever Young: Far Infrared Remineralising & Rejuvenating Seaweed Wrap Course**: Learn how to use the power of the sun, the earth & the ocean to stay young, vibrant and healthy

https://www.amazon.com/dp/B097CWDCG4

If you prefer to read books in the **PDF format**, you can buy them here:

https://purenaturecures.com/book-shop

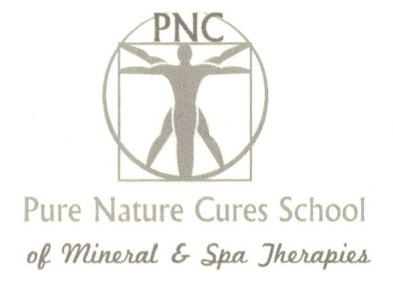

Pure Nature Cures School
of Mineral & Spa Therapies

Made in United States
Troutdale, OR
12/21/2023

16305425R00094